Perinatal Care and Considerations for Survivors of Child Abuse

Robyn Brunton • Rachel Dryer
Editors

Perinatal Care and Considerations for Survivors of Child Abuse

Challenges and Opportunities

palgrave
macmillan

Editors
Robyn Brunton
School of Psychology
Charles Sturt University
Bathurst, NSW, Australia

Rachel Dryer
School of Behavioural & Health Sciences
(Faculty of Health Science)
Australian Catholic University
Strathfield, NSW, Australia

ISBN 978-3-031-33638-6   ISBN 978-3-031-33639-3   (eBook)
https://doi.org/10.1007/978-3-031-33639-3

This Palgrave Macmillan imprint is published by the registered company Springer Nature Switzerland AG.
The registered company address is: Gewerbestrasse 11, 6330 Cham, Switzerland

Paper in this product is recyclable.

This book is dedicated to the survivors of childhood abuse. The effects of child abuse can be devasting, with wide-ranging impacts in childhood and adulthood. The life-changing developmental period of pregnancy and postpartum can bring additional challenges as individuals with this history seek to bring their own child/ren into the world. We therefore dedicate this book to you *and trust that our work will contribute to* your *empowerment and healing.*

This book is also dedicated to everyone who seeks to come alongside child abuse survivors in their perinatal journey. The clinicians, researchers, and others who provide support are driven to make this journey easier to navigate for survivors and maximize opportunities to address unresolved trauma at the right time. It is our hope that this book will contribute to improving our current practices, procedures, and policies so that optimal care and support can be provided to child abuse survivors.

The challenges and opportunities of perinatal care for child abuse survivors are best exemplified by the oft-cited nursey analogies. Fraiberg and colleagues (1975) may have shown us that ghosts in the nursery *are one of the challenges; however, it was Lieberman and colleagues' (2005)* angels in the nursery *who epitomized the opportunities.*

References

Fraiberg, S., Adelson, E., & Shapiro, V. (1975). Ghosts in the nursery. A psycho-analytic approach to the problems of impaired infant-mother relationships. Journal of the American Academy of Child Psychiatry, 14(3), 387–421. https://doi.org/10.1016/s0002-7138(09)61442-4

Lieberman, A. F., Padrón, E., Van Horn, P., & Harris, W. W. (2005). Angels in the nursery: The intergenerational transmission of benevolent parental influences. Infant Mental Health Journal, 26(6), 504–520. https://doi.org/10.1002/imhj.20071

Preface

This edited volume is a collection of current and emerging knowledge on the challenges and opportunities in the perinatal period for survivors of child abuse. The importance of this work is that it draws together research on the potential challenges that child abuse survivors may face during pregnancy and postpartum. These include, for example, mental health outcomes, childbirth difficulties, pregnancy and postpartum attachment, and intergenerational violence. We also highlight the barriers and challenges of screening for abuse and advocate for trauma-informed care and responsivity. Drawing together the research presented in the chapters of this book, we propose the Multi-level Determinants of Perinatal Well-Being for Child Abuse Survivors model as a framework for clinicians and researchers alike.

Bathurst, NSW, Australia   Robyn Brunton
Strathfield, NSW, Australia   Rachel Dryer

Acknowledgments

We sincerely thank the following people who freely gave their time and knowledge to read and provide constructive feedback on the book chapters.

Andreas Witt, Ulm University Hospital, Dr. phil. Psychologist | Child and Adolescent Psychotherapist (CBT), Head of Outpatient Psychotherapy Unit (AZVT), and Editor-in-Chief *Child and Adolescent Psychiatry and Mental Health*.

Andrew McGrath, PhD, Associate Professor at the School of Psychology, Charles Sturt University, Bathurst, NSW Australia.

Dabney Evans, PhD, MPH, Associate Professor and Director of Graduate Studies at Hubert Department of Global Health and Rollins School of Public Health Emory University.

Darryl Higgins, Professor and Director of the Institute of Child Protection Studies, Australian Catholic University, Melbourne Victoria, Australia.

Jamie Lawler, PhD, LP, Associate Professor at Eastern Michigan University.

Rachel Langevin, Assistant Professor at the Department of Educational and Counselling Psychology, McGill University.

Susan Garthus-Niegel, PhD, Dipl. Psych, Professor in Epidemiology and Women's & Family Health at the Faculty of Medicine, MSH Medical School Hamburg.

We also thank Mark Filmer, our research editor, who proofread this book and provided important and timely feedback. We also acknowledge the support of Isobel Cowper from Palgrave Macmillan, who helped bring this book to fruition.

Lastly, we want to acknowledge and thank our respective families for their continuous understanding and support of our work as researchers and educators.

About the Book

This book has a theoretical, empirical, and applied focus. Chapter 1 introduces the topic and overview of the structure of the book. Chapters 2 and 3 provide the foundation for the book with their definitional and theoretical focus. In Chap. 2, child abuse is defined, and a brief history of its conceptualization is provided, alongside prevalence and issues around assessment. These are drawn together by considering the implications for perinatal women. In Chap. 3, six theoretical perspectives are presented that offer explanations for the transactional nature of child abuse and perinatal outcomes. The psychological outcomes associated with child abuse are examined in Chaps. 4 and 5 (post-traumatic stress disorder, depression, anxiety, and suicidal thoughts and behavior). Both chapters explore the impacts of maternal child abuse on these outcomes and provide practical imperatives and directives to help address these outcomes. Chapter 6 examines specific areas of challenge across the perinatal period for survivors of child abuse. These include, for example, substance abuse and eating disorders, difficulties with motherhood and parenting, and also the challenges of childbirth. The final two chapters (7 and 8) have an applied focus. Chapter 7 considers perinatal screening and the barriers that may exist. The authors also discuss the current screening landscape and conclude with recommendations for screening to occur as part of a continuum of trauma-informed responsibility. Chapter 8, using an ecological systems approach, focuses on how to build resilience for survivors of childhood adversity. Promotive and protective factors are identified at each systems level, and the chapter also provides current interventions and strategies shown to promote resilience for perinatal women with child abuse histories. Finally, Chap. 9 draws together the research presented in the book, proposing the Multi-level Determinants of Perinatal Well-Being for Child Abuse Survivors model. This model, drawing on the research presented in the book, proposes a trauma-informed approach to screening and intervention that considers the multiple systems in which the child abuse survivor and the provider are embedded. The chapter concludes by highlighting the gaps that have been identified in research.

Contents

Notes on Contributors

Robyn Brunton, PhD. [Psych] is a Senior Lecturer at Charles Sturt University, Bathurst, NSW, Australia. Robyn has research interests in women's psychosocial health, particularly in perinatal mental health and how childhood adversity impacts women and their children in later life. More recently, Robyn has co-edited the first book on pregnancy-related anxiety with Rachel Dryer, which examines the theoretical, empirical, and clinical perspectives of this anxiety.

Rachel Dryer, PhD. [Psych] is Associate Professor of Psychology at the Australian Catholic University (Strathfield, NSW, Australia). Rachel's main research interests are in health psychology and psychological scale development. With Robyn Brunton, she co-edited the book *Pregnancy-Related Anxiety: Theory, Research, and Practice* (2021).

Teresa E. Killam is a family physician in Calgary, Alberta. She completed her medical training at the University of Calgary and residency at Women's College Hospital in Toronto. She teaches Patient Centered Care Communication Skills with the Department of Family Medicine at the University of Calgary and practices primarily low-risk obstetrics. She is also Associate Director of Student Advising and Wellness at the Cumming School of Medicine at the University of Calgary. She has championed the use of trauma-informed approaches with patients at the Riley Park

Maternity Clinic in Calgary, including leading a group of 40 family physicians to integrate the ACE questionnaire into their clinical practice.

Arianna Lane is a doctoral student in the Clinical Child Psychology PhD Program at the University of Denver. After graduating with a BA in Psychology from the University of Southern California, she spent three years coordinating research at the Children's Hospital of Los Angeles. There, she studied associations between childhood trauma and mental health in children with critical illness and the dissemination of digital interventions to improve pediatric mental health outcomes. Arianna's graduate research examines processes of risk and resilience underlying pathways between early experiences (e.g., childhood adversity and positive childhood experiences) and mental health outcomes in individuals and couples, with a particular focus on suicidal thoughts and behaviors in parents of diverse backgrounds and identities.

Sheri Madigan is a Clinical Psychologist, Professor, Canada Research Chair (Tier II), and Director of the Determinants of Child Development Lab in the Department of Psychology at the University of Calgary and the Alberta Children's Hospital Research Institute. Her research is primarily focused on understanding how children's early social experiences and relationships can influence their learning and mental health trajectories. Embedded within this work is the examination of the transmission of intergenerational risks (i.e., from parent to child), particularly the identification of mechanisms that contribute to risk, as well as resiliency factors that mitigate them.

Whitney E. Mendel is a researcher, public health educator, birth and end-of-life doula, and trauma-informed care consultant. Centering the voices and lived experiences of individuals, Whitney brings together her social work and public health roots to address systemic inequities and create trauma-informed practices, policies, and organizations.

Eva Mohler, obtained her medical degree at the University of Heidelberg Medical School and was a clinical fellow and research associate at the Department of Child and Adolescent Psychiatry, University of Heidelberg. In 2002 she became a consultant child and adolescent psychiatrist. In 2020 Eva became chair and medical director of the Child and Adolescent Psychiatric Hospital at the University of the Saarland. Her main research interests are longitudinal predictors of personality development, adverse childhood experiences, child maltreatment, and early life stress.

Angela J. Narayan is Associate Professor in the Clinical Child Psychology PhD program at the University of Denver. She received her PhD in Clinical Child Psychology from the Institute of Child Development at the University of Minnesota. She completed her APA-accredited predoctoral internship and post-doctoral fellowship in the Department of Psychiatry and Child Trauma Research Program at the University of California, San Francisco. Narayan's research focuses on the intergenerational transmission of resilience, particularly during the perinatal period, in minoritized and marginalized parents with histories of childhood adversity. She also develops empirically based methods for community mental health providers to use with underserved families. Narayan is a licensed psychologist in Colorado.

Julianna Park completed her undergraduate degree in Psychology at the University of Calgary. She is a graduate student in Clinical Psychology at Queen's University in Kingston, Ontario. Her research interests include mental, sexual, and behavioral health.

Nicole Racine is a Clinical Psychologist, Assistant Professor, and director of the Early Lab in the School of Psychology at the University of Ottawa, Canada. She holds a chair in Child and Youth Mental Health at the Children's Hospital of Eastern Ontario in Ottawa, Canada. Her research program examines the impact of maternal and childhood adversity on mental health and well-being, risk and resilience processes, and what prevention and intervention strategies break cycles of risk across generations.

Julia Seng, PhD, RN, CNM, FACNM, FAAN is a nurse-midwife and Professor of Nursing, Obstetrics & Gynecology, and Women's and Gender Studies at the University of Michigan. Her program of research has applied qualitative, clinical, and biobehavioral approaches focusing on the effects of maltreatment-related posttraumatic stress on perinatal, maternal mental health, and early parenting outcomes of trauma survivors. She is a co-developer with Mickey Sperlich, PhD, MSW, CPM, of the *Survivor Moms' Companion*, a perinatal trauma-specific intervention for childbearing people with a history of childhood maltreatment. She partners with end-user organizations to study the implementation of the *Survivor Moms' Companion* program.

Mickey Sperlich is an experienced midwife and researcher who studies the effects of trauma and mental health challenges related to reproduction. She is co-creator of a psychosocial intervention for pregnant survivors of abuse and is committed to developing transdisciplinary approaches to address the sequelae of sexual violence and other trauma.

Cassandra Svelnys is a doctoral student in the Clinical Child Psychology PhD Program at the University of Denver. She received her BA in Psychology from the University of Connecticut and her MA in Clinical Child Psychology from the University of Denver. Prior to her doctoral training, Cassandra worked as a clinical research specialist at Boston Children's Hospital. Cassandra's research focuses on understanding intergenerational pathways of trauma and resilience, with a particular focus on the effects of child maltreatment. Cassandra's work also emphasizes community-engaged research that includes centering individuals' lived experiences, values, and knowledge in empirically based methods, particularly within marginalized and underserved communities.

About the Editors

Robyn Brunton is a Senior Lecturer with the School of Psychology at Charles Sturt University (Bathurst, NSW, Australia). Robyn's research interest is in women's psychosocial health, particularly health and well-being during pregnancy. This is the second book that Robyn has co-edited, with the first a collective examination of theory, research, and clinical perspectives of pregnancy-related anxiety.

Rachel Dryer is Associate Professor of Psychology in the School of Behavioural and Health Sciences at the Australian Catholic University (Strathfield, NSW, Australia). Rachel is a registered psychologist whose research interests are in health psychology, particularly women's mental health during pregnancy and post-partum, body image, and disordered eating behaviors. Rachel also has a key interest in psychological scale development.

List of Figures

List of Tables

1

Introduction

Robyn Brunton (iD)

Abstract This first chapter provides an overview of the book, laying out its theoretical, empirical, and applied structure. Theoretically, the importance of studying child abuse is discussed, and theories that provide the explanatory power of maternal experiences for survivors are provided. Empirically, psychological outcomes are examined that include post-traumatic stress disorder, depression, anxiety, and suicidal thoughts using a developmental pathway perspective. Other challenges for survivors that have drawn a particular focus in the literature, including eating disorders, motherhood-child bonding, and childbirth, are examined. The final chapters provide an applied perspective considering the challenges and opportunities afforded by screening, with a focus on trauma-informed care and strategies for building resilience for survivors of childhood adversity. Finally, drawing on the research in the book, the Multi-level Determinants of Perinatal Well-Being for Child Abuse Survivors model

R. Brunton (✉)
School of Psychology, Charles Sturt University, Bathurst, NSW, Australia
e-mail: rbrunton@csu.edu.au

© The Author(s), under exclusive license to Springer Nature Switzerland AG 2023
R. Brunton, R. Dryer (eds.), *Perinatal Care and Considerations for Survivors of Child Abuse*, https://doi.org/10.1007/978-3-031-33639-3_1

is proposed, providing a framework for clinicians to provide a trauma-informed care for survivors. The chapter concludes by asserting that the book, with its focus on areas that intersect between clinicians, researchers, and psychologists, will be a valuable resource for professionals in this area.

Keywords Child abuse • Child maltreatment • Perinatal challenges • Psychopathology • Resilience • Screening

Pregnancy, childbirth, and the first year of motherhood (i.e., the perinatal period) are profound and life-changing events impacting all areas of a woman's life (Issokson, 2004; Lederman & Weis, 2009). This normative developmental period can be depicted as joyous and a time to blossom, but for some women who are survivors of child abuse (i.e., physical, sexual, psychological, or emotional abuse), it can be particularly challenging. This challenge can come from the intersectionality of the impact of maternal experiences of child abuse and the universal tasks of pregnancy, which may be more difficult for survivors. For example, acceptance is one of the first psychological tasks of pregnancy (Lederman & Weis, 2009), which may be difficult to achieve with ongoing doubts about bringing a child into a world perceived as unsafe for children, based on the mother's abusive history, despite the desire for a baby (Issokson, 2004). Also, the physical experience of pregnancy, which can include morning sickness, weight gain, and a changing body shape, can lead to feelings of a lack of control of the body, which can be triggering for abuse survivors. Childbirth and its associated intimate procedures, which may be standard practice in prenatal care, can feel intrusive and anxiety-provoking for survivors (Issokson, 2004). Postpartum, many survivors report pain, disassociation, and anxiety when breastfeeding (Coles et al., 2016), and for some, the normative arousal experienced or lack of success with breastfeeding can induce shame, guilt, and feelings of failure (Issokson, 2004), making this a challenging experience. Thus, the perinatal period can be fraught with challenges for survivors of child abuse.

Given these considerations, pregnancy and postpartum can also present unique challenges for clinicians and mental health professionals.

These include antenatal care considerations, such as triggering events (e.g., intimate procedures) that can re-traumatize women or result in avoidance of routine care. Other associated adverse outcomes include increased health concerns (e.g., more significant somatic complaints), prolonged labor, and preterm birth. However, these challenges also present opportunities through interventions and resilience building. Differential outcomes of child abuse suggest that some women are more resilient to the potential impacts of child abuse than others. However, issues around disclosure of abuse may mean that some clinicians and mental health professionals are unaware that the women in their care are child abuse survivors. This suggests that consideration of more universal precautions, such as trauma-informed care, may be needed.

This book draws together research concerning these challenges and opportunities during the perinatal period for survivors of child abuse. While this book provides a focused examination of child abuse and how it may impact perinatal women, we acknowledge that childhood neglect can also have far-reaching consequences. However, our focus on child abuse is particularly important as different types of abuse are known to have differential outcomes for perinatal women. In addition, the child abuse subtypes also have distinct characteristics and associated behaviors that can have differential impacts during pregnancy and postpartum. Therefore, it is essential to understand these implications for perinatal care. This book provides a broad-stroke approach by considering topics ranging from psychological challenges during pregnancy to a detailed discussion on screening and resilience. In addition, this book adds to the existing body of knowledge by pulling together the current and emerging literature on perinatal outcomes for child abuse survivors drawing on empirical findings and theory.

The chapters in the book have a theoretical (Chaps. 2 and 3), empirical (Chaps. 4, 5, and 6), and applied (Chaps. 7 and 8) focus. Specifically, Chap. 2 provides definitions of child abuse, how it has been conceptualized historically, and the prevalence of child abuse, and highlights key issues around the assessment of abuse and implications for perinatal women. The chapter also examines the importance of assessing and controlling for the different abuse types, providing a more detailed understanding of the associated challenges and opportunities for perinatal women. The theoretical perspectives outlined and examined in Chap. 3 offer explanatory power in relation to maternal experiences of child abuse, and all account for the transactional nature of abuse experiences and perinatal outcomes. Together Chaps. 2 and 3 provide an essential foundation for the book.

Chapters 4 and 5 examine psychological outcomes associated with abuse. Chapter 4 examines childbearing through a post-traumatic stress disorder (PTSD) lens, including the challenges associated with childbirth, such as intrusive and recurring memories of abuse and normative childbirth experiences that may be triggering for some. The chapter also explores the role of perinatal providers in addressing PTSD and implores us to address unresolved trauma ahead of parenting and to provide care that resists re-traumatization. Chapter 5 builds on this psychological focus by examining three mental health problems that can be experienced during the perinatal period. By applying a developmental psychopathology perspective, the pathways from childhood abuse to depression, anxiety, and suicidal thoughts and behavior are examined. The chapter describes intervening mechanisms (e.g., emotion dysregulation) implicated in these pathways and examines the issue of comorbidity. Finally, the chapter concludes with a directive to improve understanding of the effects of early life adversities and mental health problems in gender-diverse pregnant individuals.

Chapter 6 discusses pertinent areas that have drawn particular focus in the literature that may be challenging across the perinatal period. First, general and psychological health and their implications for mother and child are considered. This includes related issues, such as prenatal substance abuse and eating disorders, which have implications for the developing fetus. The chapter then examines motherhood, particularly mother-child bonding, an essential aspect of motherhood that has been shown to develop far earlier (during pregnancy) than first thought. Relatedly, the challenges associated with breastfeeding (important for attachment and bonding) for child abuse survivors are considered. Finally, this part of the chapter ends with parenting and the difficulties potentially encountered by child abuse survivors, such as hostile parenting behavior and a lack of emotional availability. The last part of this chapter examines intergenerational abuse and childbirth. The higher risk of revictimization for child abuse survivors has implications for mother and child, with the associated stress or physical harm potentially contributing to preterm birth, miscarriage, and, in extreme cases, mortality. Childbirth studies confirm that the experience of childbirth can present a particular challenge for survivors; however, positive birth experiences provide an opportunity to attenuate the impact of abuse history in subsequent pregnancies.

Chapter 7 considers perinatal screening for child abuse and trauma. Barriers to screening are also considered, including irregular screening practices, clinician discomfort, fear of causing distress, and inadequate support and referral services. The screening landscape is next considered, concluding that current recommendations are piecemeal with related risk factors (e.g., mood disorders) screened in isolation. Indeed, screening for child abuse is not routinely done, suggesting the need for comprehensive psychosocial assessment. Finally, the chapter provides recommendations for screening as part of a continuum of trauma-informed responsivity across all levels of practice. Basic recommendations and precautions across contexts are offered, including recommendations for responsivity in the absence of disclosure and considerations of the clinician's history of trauma.

Chapter 8 is focused on building resilience for survivors of childhood adversity in the perinatal period. Using an ecological systems approach, the chapter provides an overview of the individual-, family-, community-, and systems-level factors that can alter or affect the association between child abuse and maternal mental health. Promotive and protective factors that play a role in resilience are identified for each level. At an individual level, these include self-esteem, positive attribution styles, and coping. Family-level factors include parenting relationships and perceptions of security and safety. Community- and system-level factors include social networks, support, and cultural and environmental backgrounds. The chapter identifies current interventions and resilience-promoting strategies that have efficacy for perinatal women with child abuse histories, providing details of specific programs that aim to promote adaptive mental health and parenting outcomes at different ecological levels. Drawing on the research in the book, the authors propose the Multi-level Determinants of Perinatal Well-Being for Child Abuse Survivors model.

This model provides a useful framework for clinicians to provide a trauma-informed care for survivors. The chapter concludes by identifying the need for further research within the perinatal setting to advance the understanding of how to build resilience in the perinatal period for survivors of childhood abuse and adversity.

This book will be a valuable resource for professionals caring for perinatal women by focusing on areas that intersect between clinicians (midwives), researchers, and psychologists. By bringing these disciplines together, we offer a thorough and in-depth assessment of child abuse, pregnancy, and postpartum with a theoretical, empirical, and applied focus. We trust that this book will assist professionals who need a primary source to advance their knowledge and understanding of the literature, current issues, and implications for clinical practice and future research concerning child abuse and perinatal women.

References

Coles, J., Anderson, A., & Loxton, D. (2016). Breastfeeding duration after childhood sexual abuse: An Australian cohort study. *Journal of Human Lactation,* *32*(3), NP28–NP35. https://doi.org/10.1177/089033441 5590782

Issokson, D. (2004). *Effects of childhood abuse on childbearing and perinatal health.* American Psychological Association.

Lederman, R. P., & Weis, K. (2009). *Psychosocial adaptation to pregnancy; seven dimensions of maternal role development* (3rd ed.). Springer.

2

Child Abuse: Definitions, Prevalence, and Considerations in Assessment

Robyn Brunton 🆔

Abstract This chapter discusses the wide variability in conceptualizations and definitions of child abuse over time and cross-culturally. Commonly recognized forms of child abuse are physical and sexual; psychological and emotional abuse are less recognized, with variability in the relatedness of these types. Examinations of child abuse and maltreatment more broadly show that survivors may be more likely to experience adverse perinatal outcomes. However, a key limitation of the research is a failure to examine differential associations and a focus on child sexual abuse. Given the distinct characteristics of abuse types, understanding their potential differential impact on perinatal women is important for providing evidence-based care. The assessment of abuse also differs, with child abuse not always a single event but rather an ongoing pattern of victimization. Multitype maltreatment recognizes this and also the interconnectedness of maltreatment experiences. The adverse childhood experiences (ACEs) approach is commonly used, recognizing a range of

R. Brunton (✉)
School of Psychology, Charles Sturt University, Bathurst, NSW, Australia
e-mail: rbrunton@csu.edu.au

adversity (abuse and dysfunction); however, it is criticized as a simplistic representation of adverse experiences, particularly given the equivalent risk it assumes for each experience. For pregnant/postpartum women, research into the abuse subtypes provides a more detailed understanding of the challenges and opportunities in perinatal care. Given the prevalence of abuse worldwide, the likelihood that an expectant mother will be a child abuse survivor is high. Child abuse can have serious and wideranging implications for perinatal women; therefore, understanding their needs is essential to working toward optimal outcomes for both mother and child.

Keywords Child abuse and perinatal outcomes • Abuse and pregnancy • Abuse and postpartum

Worldwide, millions of children are impacted by child abuse and neglect (i.e., maltreatment), with research confirming long-term deleterious outcomes (Souch et al., 2022; Strathearn et al., 2020). The breadth of concern for this adversity is demonstrated by the World Health Organization, calling for the global recognition of child maltreatment as a public health concern (Arie, 2005). Child maltreatment is an overarching term encompassing all types of child abuse and other forms of maltreatment, such as child exploitation and trafficking (Leeb et al., 2008). In contrast, child abuse includes specific abusive acts perpetrated in childhood. These acts can be physical, sexual, psychological, or emotional. Often, child abuse and child maltreatment are used interchangeably; however, an important distinction is that child abuse refers to the commission of intentional and unintentional acts (e.g., punishment with unintended consequences). Conversely, child maltreatment includes neglect (the omission of certain acts, such as a failure to provide adequate care) and other harmful behaviors (Leeb et al., 2008).

This chapter will define child abuse, provide background on the identification of child abuse and key issues around assessing child abuse, and highlight the implications for perinatal women. By drawing on empirical research, the chapter provides background for the subsequent chapters in this book.

Why Just Child Abuse?

Child abuse and neglect in the general population, and for perinatal women specifically, can have differential outcomes (Lang et al., 2010; Souch et al., 2022). Pregnant women with a child abuse or maltreatment history are at greater risk of adverse perinatal outcomes, such as miscarriage (Abajobir et al., 2018), postpartum depression (Giallo et al., 2017), and preterm birth (Selk et al., 2016) than women with no such history. Often these associations are stronger for certain abuse subtypes (e.g., forced sexual activity, but not physical abuse, is associated with preterm birth, Selk et al., 2016); however, the propensity to examine maltreatment in general, without examination of the subtypes of abuse, may limit our understanding.

Moreover, within the perinatal literature when subtypes of abuse are considered, historically, research has focused more on child sexual abuse. Women with a maternal history of child sexual abuse, for example, can have greater childbirth concerns or fear feeling powerless, and for some, pregnancy is the first-time memories of their abuse resurface (Leeners et al., 2016). Moreover, intimate medical procedures associated with their care can create distress and, in some cases, lead to flashbacks, disassociation, and other post-traumatic stress disorder (PTSD)-like symptoms and avoidance of prenatal care (Issokson, 2004; Leeners et al., 2007). For women with maternal child sexual abuse, their experience of pregnancy and childbirth is often negative and more frightening compared to other women (Brunton, 2021; Leeners et al., 2016). While this focus on child sexual abuse is understandable given the obvious links between the experience of this abuse and the associated tasks of pregnancy, the extent to which other abuse types may make the experiences of pregnancy and postpartum more challenging is less studied, despite being equally important to know.

The importance of subtype analysis is further supported by the distinct characteristics and associated behaviors of the different abuse types. That is, the experience of sexual abuse differs from that of emotional or physical abuse. The impact of these behaviorally distinct aspects of abuse is important to understand in the context of pregnancy and postpartum.

However, only a handful of studies examine specific abuse subtypes in the perinatal literature. For example, two studies identified maternal childhood physical abuse or corporal punishment (with physical damage) as risk factors for child abuse potential, which is the capacity for mothers to become perpetrators of child abuse (De Paúl & Domenech, 2000; Ornduff et al., 2002). Conversely, others have found that women who suffered emotional/psychological abuse during childhood may have more difficulty with internal representations of motherhood, an important developmental task of pregnancy, potentially impacting maternal-fetal or mother-infant attachment (Chap. 6 provides an overview). Yet of 49 studies identified in a recent review of child maltreatment and perinatal outcomes, only 22 examined specific subtypes of child abuse. The authors concluded that without subtype analysis, relationships between these adversities and perinatal outcomes are poorly understood (Souch et al., 2022). Given the uniqueness of pregnancy as a developmental life stage, certain triggers or sensitivities can exacerbate perinatal outcomes. However, our knowledge of the differential impacts of child abuse may be limited, and this could have implications for providing evidence-based perinatal care.

Historical Background of Child Abuse

Child abuse is not a new phenomenon and has occurred throughout history (Newberger et al., 1982), yet its recognition is more recent. Approximately 150 years ago, a landmark legal case involved the American Society for the Prevention of Cruelty to Animals acting for an abused child, being the only agency willing and available to do so (Solomon, 1973). This case and the accompanying public outcry were cataclysmic in formally recognizing child abuse and establishing appropriate services in the United States of America. Despite this, it was not until the 1960s that Henry Kempe identified the *battered-child syndrome* (Kempe et al., 1985, p. 143) to "characterize a clinical condition in young children" who were seriously physically abused. This abuse, Kempe noted, was usually perpetrated by their caregiver and not dependent on personality or socioeconomic status but rather occurred among all people regardless of education and socioeconomic status.

In contrast, child sexual abuse was considered rare before the late 1970s and emerged as a social and public issue[1] through the child protection and feminist movements (Finkelhor, 1979; Putnam, 2003). Child protection advocates viewed child sexual abuse as part of the battered-child syndrome, which likely contributed to child physical and sexual abuse, often viewed as one phenomenon (Finkelhor, 1979). Conversely, the feminist movement saw child sexual abuse as a subcategory of adult sexual assault. Despite these differences, these movements brought the issue of child sexual abuse to the fore (Finkelhor, 1979). With the introduction of official statistics, the incidence of child sexual abuse seemed to increase dramatically, with studies in the 1980s–1990s reporting the prevalence as high as 62%. Yet the wide variability in the definitions, age limits, and measures used contributed to the disparity in the numbers reported (Finkelhor, 1994). Regardless, this perceived increase in the reported prevalence likely contributed to the growing awareness of this social and public issue.

Historically, physical and sexual abuse have received more clinical and research attention than psychological or emotional abuse. This focus is likely due to physical and sexual abuse being more 'tangible,' with disclosure often constituting a crisis (O'Hagan, 1993). On the other hand, psychological/emotional abuse is less obvious, sometimes more challenging to articulate for the victim, and often inherent in other abusive or neglectful acts (Ferguson & Dacey, 1997; O'Hagan, 1993). Indeed, there is a strong argument that psychological/emotional abuse is inherent in all abuse types (Cawson et al., 2000; Ferguson & Dacey, 1997).

---

[1] Social problems are situations recognized by some of the population, whereas a public issue is one recognized by a broad section of society. Not all social issues become public issues (Finkelhor, 1979).

Defining Child Abuse

Given the many different contexts and ways in which children can be harmed, defining child abuse is challenging (Cawson et al., 2000). In most developed countries, child abuse is considered to be acts against a child or young person that are physical, sexual, emotional, or psychological (ACT Parliamentary Counsel, 2022). While child abuse definitions generally focus on these acts, many definitions fail to consider cross-cultural differences in what constitutes child abuse.

The most recognized types of child abuse are physical and sexual (IPSCAN, 2008).[2] A survey of 23 developed countries[3] showed agreement that physical abuse, sexual abuse, and neglect constitute child maltreatment, with less consensus for emotional abuse or psychological neglect. Of the 52 developing countries surveyed, most agreed (96.2%) that sexual abuse was abusive, with fewer acknowledging physical abuse (5.8%). This lack of recognition of physical abuse can stem from parenting practices that may be acceptable in one culture but considered abusive in others (AIFS, 2018). For example, child physical abuse is rarely recognized in China as it is considered child discipline or domestic violence (Qiao & Chan, 2005). Therefore, these cross-cultural variations in conceptualizations of abuse contribute to global inconsistencies.

Another point of difference is definitions derived for different purposes. The broader legal definitions contrast with more detailed definitions used for research, intervention, and treatment (AIFS, 2018; Australian Law Reform Commission, 2022). These broader and more detailed definitions can create inconsistencies as often, within the detail, disagreement exists. In addition, age limits that define 'child' are often aligned with the age of consent, which can vary widely among countries, ranging from 11 years in Nigeria to 21 years in Bahrain (Hulme, 2004, provides a fuller discussion; World Population Review, 2022). Moreover, some child sexual abuse studies include a 5-year age qualifier between the

---

[2] Based on information from 75 countries, of which 52 (or 69%) were considered developing countries.

[3] Countries with low and lower-middle incomes were classified as developing; countries with upper-middle and high incomes were classified as developed.

perpetrator and victim to exclude sex play or exploration (Hulme, 2004). These issues complicate research and clinical work by inhibiting the creation of a body of research based on a strong definitional foundation. A recent systematic review highlighted the inconsistencies around these definitions, age limits, and qualifiers. The authors proposed that removing the age limit and placing the determination "on the survivor's perception (i.e., I believe I was sexually abused as a child)" would contribute to consistency and allay concerns about including consensual acts (Brunton & Dryer, 2021, p. 12).

Definitions of Abuse Types

While child abuse is a broad term, four main abuse types are commonly recognized. Table 2.1 provides definitions. As shown, child physical abuse refers to the commission or omission of certain acts that cause harm and is considered the most studied type of abuse in the general population (Arata et al., 2005; Higgins & McCabe, 2001).

Despite recent child maltreatment studies being dominated by child sexual abuse (Stoltenborgh et al., 2015), there is little consensus on what behaviors constitute it or the age that delineates a child from an adult (Haugaard, 2000). The definition for child sexual abuse provided below is broader than other definitions (e.g., see the definitions provided by IPSCAN, 2008, p. 52), recognizing the breadth of abusive acts, cultural differences, and informed consent.

Psychological abuse relates to the cognitive appraisal of certain acts. In contrast, emotional abuse focuses more on behavior that can harm the child's experience and expression of emotion. Psychological and emotional abuse are often used interchangeably or considered synonymous, which likely emanates from emotion and cognition, generally considered to be interdependent (AIFS, 2018; O'Hagan, 1995; Robinson, 2019). Garbarino (1989, p. 502)[4] defines psychological maltreatment as "a concerted attack on the development of self and social competence, an assault on the psyche" and proposes psychological maltreatment in terms of five

---

[4] The title 'The Psychologically Battered Child' is an acknowledgment of Kempe's initial work in identifying abused children (Garbarino, 2013).

Table 2.1 Child abuse definitions

Abuse type	Definition
Physical	Physical acts against a child that are perpetrated by a parent or caregiver, or the omission of acts that protect a child from physical abuse. These acts include hitting with a body part or weapon (such as a stick or belt), kicking, punching, shoving, throwing the child, dragging and dropping, shaking, choking, burning, and poisoning. (Mathews et al., 2021; Robinson, 2019, p. 13)
Sexual	Both contact or non-contact sexual activity that violates the standards of the relevant society. These acts are by anyone in a position of power over the child and used for sexual gratification. The child does not fully understand, is not developmentally prepared, cannot provide consent, or does not consent if capable. (Mathews et al., 2021; WHO, 1999, Appendix A)
Psychological	Intentional behavior (e.g., blaming, belittling, or isolating) that is continual (e.g., chronic) or episodic (e.g., triggered by a specific context or situation) that conveys that a child is worthless, flawed, unloved, unwanted, endangered, or valued only in meeting another's needs. (Leeb et al., 2008, p. 16)
Emotional	Failure to provide a developmentally appropriate, supportive environment for the development of a stable and full range of emotional and social competencies according to the child's personal potential and in the context of the society in which the child develops. (WHO, 1999, Appendix A)

categories that include both psychological and emotional components. These include rejecting, isolating (excluding the child socially), terrorizing (verbal assault, creating fear), ignoring (depriving the child of essential stimulation and responsiveness, emotional starvation), and corrupting (mis-socializing the child).

Prevalence of Child Abuse

Prevalence estimates of child abuse vary dramatically (e.g., 0–90%, Stoltenborgh et al., 2015). While some variability may reflect actual differences in the occurrence of this phenomenon, a large proportion relates to issues highlighted above relating to definition and measurement.

Moreover, estimates from reported incidents of child abuse are considered conservative, as not all incidents are reported. Many victims of abuse never disclose their experiences or do so many years later. Therefore, administrative data such as from child protection agencies do not provide a complete picture and likely represent a small proportion of abuse experiences in the population (Mathews et al., 2016).

A recent review (Moody et al., 2018) aimed to establish the prevalence of the different types of child maltreatment globally.[5] This comprehensive review of 337 articles included retrospective self-reports of child maltreatment (under 18 years) from studies published from 2000 onward. Given our perinatal focus, we only report the prevalence for girls in Table 2.2. As shown, wide variability exists across global regions, with higher estimates drawn from smaller study samples (i.e., Australia, South America). Indeed, in Australia, there has been limited comprehensive assessment of child abuse at the population level (Mathews et al., 2021). Further, differing conceptions of abuse contribute to the variability shown. Therefore, these estimates should be cautiously interpreted.

Notwithstanding the inconsistencies in prevalence, there is no doubt that child abuse is a worldwide phenomenon. Also, given the above prevalence estimates and the approximate 140 million births per annum (The World Counts, 2022), a significant proportion of perinatal women will

Table 2.2 Prevalence of abuse types for girls only; the median is reported with the number of studies in parentheses

Abuse type	North America	South America	Asia	Europe	Africa	Australia
Physical	21.7% (78)	59.0% (2)	22.8% (20)	12.0% (11)	50.8% (6)	53.4% (1)
Sexual	20.4% (106)	22.4% (2)	9.0% (43)	14.3% (27)	18.9 (14)	28.8% (12)
Emotional or psychological	28.4% (32)	60.0% (2)	26.9% (14)	12.9% (8)	30.5% (2)	55.9% (1)

[5] We make the observation that most studies in reporting prevalence are actually reporting incidence or occurrence. The term incidence or occurrence refers to cases of abuse that occurred within a specified period, and prevalence refers to the percentage of children victimized by such an experience, and this could be once or many times (Russell, 1984).

have a child abuse history. In one study of 638 pregnant women, over 60% reported at least one instance of physical, sexual, or psychological childhood abuse (Brunton et al., 2020).

Assessing Child Abuse and Maltreatment

Multitype Maltreatment

For many children, abuse is not a single event but part of an ongoing pattern of victimization (Finkelhor et al., 2007). Research shows that previous abuse is a risk factor for ongoing or other child abuse (Boney-McCoy & Finkelhor, 1995; Radford et al., 2011), and findings such as these have turned the focus to multi-type maltreatment (Price-Robertson et al., 2013). Multi-type maltreatment recognizes the interconnectedness of maltreatment experiences and its high comorbidity for many individuals (Higgins & McCabe, 2001). However, historically, child abuse studies have primarily focused on single abuse types (Arata et al., 2005; Dong et al., 2004). While different abuse types do not always co-occur, with studies reporting varying correlations between abuse types ranging from low to high (Clemmons et al., 2007; Higgins & McCabe, 2001; Matsumoto et al., 2020), the probability that they do occur simultaneously or consecutively is high. For example, emotional and psychological abuse are more likely to be experienced in any abuse (Cawson et al., 2000), and the experience of sexual abuse may often involve physical abuse (Higgins & McCabe, 2001). Thus, it is important that when examining abuse, the effects of other types of abuse or maltreatment are statistically controlled.

This statistical control (i.e., partitioning the effects of other abuse types statistically, such as controlling for other abuses when examining physical abuse) provides a more comprehensive assessment of child abuse. Failure to include other abuse or maltreatment types within these statistical models limits the ability to determine the specific effect of a type of abuse (Higgins & McCabe, 2001) and may inflate particular findings. Given the high probability that abuse experiences will be comorbid, not doing so can impinge on our understanding (see Higgins & McCabe, 2001, for a comprehensive review).

Research also shows that experiencing multiple instances of maltreatment is linked to poorer outcomes (Arata et al., 2005; Clemmons et al., 2007). These findings suggest that survivors who have experienced a greater frequency or severity of abuse may be at risk of poorer outcomes than those subjected to single abuse experiences. However, many studies examine abuse dichotomously; that is, they assess the occurrence of abuse (yes or no), but not the frequency of abuse as a continuous variable. Regarding pregnancy and childbirth, findings show that as the severity or frequency of abuse increases, so do the adverse outcomes. Many studies show a dose-response relationship (e.g., Brunton et al., 2020; Gelaye et al., 2015; Zhang et al., 2020). Therefore, this approach may also limit our understanding.

Adverse Childhood Experiences

One such measure that uses a similar approach is the commonly used adverse childhood experiences (ACEs) questionnaire. The ACEs questionnaire was initially developed to investigate the association between childhood adversity and adult health risk and disease (Felitti et al., 1998). ACEs are typically assessed by a retrospective questionnaire on the occurrence of physical abuse, sexual abuse, psychological abuse, and household dysfunction (i.e., exposure to substance abuse, mental illness, violent treatment of mother or stepmother, and criminal behavior) before the age of 18 years (Felitti et al., 1998). Each exposure category is scored dichotomously. Since its original publication, several versions and revisions of the ACEs questionnaire have been published (see Asmussen et al., 2020 for a review), and it is now a common means of assessing child abuse and household dysfunction. The ACEs summary score, which is the sum of the number of exposures per category (e.g., physical abuse), provides an ordinal measure of child abuse (Dong et al., 2004).

Research using the ACEs questionnaire has been prolific and increased awareness of the lifetime impact of early adversity (Lacey & Minnis, 2020). Notwithstanding this, the ACEs approach has been criticized as simplistic and disregarding the complexity of child abuse and maltreatment (Lacey & Minnis, 2020). ACEs assume an equal impact of each adverse experience, and thus apportion an equivalent risk (Lanier et al., 2018). Indeed, the ACEs have been called "an overly simplified representation" of these experiences (Ford et al., 2014, p. 441). To address this limitation, studies have adapted the ACEs to assess the frequency of abuse (e.g., Brunton et al., 2020), providing a more nuanced assessment. However, despite this, many studies still use the ACE summary score to assess maternal experiences of abuse (e.g., Nidey et al., 2020).

Implications for Perinatal Women

It is important to note that not all child abuse victims suffer long-term adverse effects (Collishaw et al., 2007). However, some individuals experience various deleterious outcomes. These include neurological changes, direct injuries from the abuse, ongoing health consequences (e.g., failure to thrive, obesity), increased risk of disease (e.g., asthma), psychological outcomes (e.g., attachment issues, externalizing and internalizing behaviors), and PTSD (see Leeb et al., 2011 for a review).

One of the first published articles highlighting that pregnancy and childbirth can be re-traumatizing for abuse survivors was Anna Rose's honest and confronting account of her pregnancy and birth experience (Rose, 1992). The publication of this article was consistent with the growing recognition of the impact of child abuse on pregnancy emanating from the public and social events discussed above. Early attention was focused on abuse as a risk factor for teen pregnancy (see Donaldson et al., 1989, for example), with studies confirming that child sexual abuse increased the odds of experiencing adolescent pregnancy (Adams & East, 1999; Logan et al., 2007). Attention was also focused on the sequelae of child sexual abuse specific to childbirth (Rhodes & Hutchinson, 1994), pregnancy and birth behaviors (Grimstad & Schei, 1999), and perinatal care (Courtois & Courtois Riley, 1992). Research consistently confirmed that child sexual abuse was associated with poorer outcomes in these areas.

More recently, within the perinatal literature, the focus on child sexual abuse has been renewed with studies examining the birthing experience (e.g., Heimstad et al., 2006; Leeners et al., 2016; Lukasse et al., 2010). For many survivors, childbirth is re-traumatizing (Melender, 2002), with key findings including that pregnant women with this history may express a preference for a cesarean, experience greater fear of childbirth, and, in some cases, disassociate due to the prior abusive experiences (see Brunton, 2021 for a review).

Research into the implications for survivors of child sexual abuse is important. Still, there needs to be greater consideration for all child abuse survivors, as their experiences and potential sequelae may impact their perinatal care. Moreover, considering that physical abuse is usually the most common abuse type experienced, overlooking the implications of specific abuse types represents a potential knowledge gap. For example, child abuse presents a particular risk for re-victimization in adulthood (Barnett et al., 2018). Research indicates differential associations depending on the type of childhood abuse and re-victimization. For example, child sexual abuse and/or child physical abuse are stronger risk factors for physical and/or sexual intimate partner violence (IPV). In contrast, the risk of experiencing emotional IPV is over fourfold for child emotional abuse survivors, with lower odds for child physical or sexual abuse and revictimization. In studies that examined IPV overall, psychological and sexual abuse were the only significant predictors; each independently increased the risk around fourfold (LoCascio et al., 2018). Pregnancy is a time of particular vulnerability for IPV (Campo, 2015), which suggests that being a child abuse survivor and pregnant, likely increases the risk of IPV exponentially. Therefore, understanding the risk of different abuse types is important, particularly in tailoring effective interventions for IPV. While these findings relate only to IPV specifically, it is conceivable that these differential outcomes exist for other areas and abuse types. Without further research, this, unfortunately, remains unclear.

Conclusion

This chapter discussed child abuse, its history, definitions, prevalence, and assessment. As can be seen, over the past decades, our understanding of child abuse and its potential sequelae has increased. However, there is still much to learn. While in the general population, child physical abuse commands attention, within the perinatal literature, the tendency is to focus on child sexual abuse. This focus is grounded in good reasons, given that this childhood adversity can present challenges for pregnant and postpartum women. Yet, we limit our understanding of the impact of child abuse by failing to account for the comorbidity or assuming equivalency of risk. Also, without disentangling the effects of particular abuse types or assessing frequency/severity, it limits our understanding of perinatal women. The perinatal period presents great change and adjustment for women and can be a particular time of vulnerability for child abuse survivors. Therefore, it is imperative for researchers to extend our understanding of the needs of women who are survivors of child abuse to ensure optimal outcomes for both mother and child.

References

Abajobir, A. A., Kisely, S., Williams, G., Strathearn, L., & Najman, J. M. (2018). Risky sexual behaviors and pregnancy outcomes in young adulthood following substantiated childhood maltreatment: Findings from a prospective birth cohort study. *The Journal of Sex Research, 55*(1), 106–119. https://doi.org/1 0.1080/00224499.2017.1368975

ACT Parliamentary Counsel. (2022). *Children and Young People Act 2008*. www. legislation.act.gov.au

Adams, J. A., & East, P. (1999). Past physical abuse is significantly correlated with pregnancy as an adolescent. *Journal of Pediatric and Adolescent Gynecology, 12*(3), 133–138. https://doi.org/10.1016/s1038-3188(99)00005-4

AIFS. (2018). *What is child abuse and neglect?* https://aifs.gov.au/cfca/publications/what-child-abuse-and-neglect

Arata, C. M., Langhinrichsen-Rohling, J., Bowers, D., & O'Farrill-Swails, L. (2005). Single versus multi-type maltreatment. *Journal of Aggression, Maltreatment & Trauma, 11*(4), 29–52. https://doi.org/10.1300/J146v11n04_02

Arie, S. (2005). WHO takes up issue of child abuse. *BMJ: British Medical Journal, 331*(7509), 129. https://doi.org/10.1136/bmj.331.7509.129

Asmussen, K., Fischer, F., Drayton, E., & McBride, T. (2020). *Adverse childhood experiences: What we know, what we don't know, and what should happen next.*

https://www.eif.org.uk/report/adverse-childhoodexperiences-what-we-know-what-we-dont-know-and-whatshould-happen-next

Australian Law Reform Commission. (2022). *Criminal offences relating to child protection.* https://www.alrc.gov.au/publication/family-violence-a-national-legal-response-alrc-report-114/20-family-violence-child-protection-and-the-criminal-law-3/criminal-offences-relating-to-child-protection/

Barnett, W., Halligan, S., Heron, J., Fraser, A., Koen, N., Zar, H. J., Donald, K. A., & Stein, D. J. (2018). Maltreatment in childhood and intimate partner violence: A latent class growth analysis in a South African pregnancy cohort. *Child Abuse & Neglect, 86,* 336–348. https://doi.org/10.1016/j.chiabu.2018.08.020

Boney-McCoy, S., & Finkelhor, D. (1995). Prior victimization: A risk factor for child sexual abuse and for PTSD-related symptomatology among sexually abused youth. *Child Abuse & Neglect, 19*(12), 1401–1421. https://doi.org/10.1016/0145-2134(95)00104-9

Brunton, R. (2021). Psychosocial functioning and sexual abuse. In R. Dryer & R. Brunton (Eds.), *Pregnancy-related anxiety: Research, theory and practice.* Routledge.

Brunton, R., & Dryer, R. (2021). Child sexual abuse and pregnancy: A systematic review of the literature. *Child Abuse & Neglect, 111,* 104802. https://doi.org/10.1016/j.chiabu.2020.104802

Brunton, R., Wood, T., & Dryer, R. (2020). Childhood abuse, pregnancy-related anxiety and the mediating role of resilience and social support. *The Journal of Health Psychology, 1359105320968140,* 868. https://doi.org/10.1177/1359105320968140

Campo, M. (2015). *Domestic and family violence in pregnancy and early parenthood.* Australian Institute of Family Studies. https://apo.org.au/node/61040

Cawson, P., Wattam, C., Brooker, S., & Kelly, G. (2000). *Child maltreatment in the United Kingdom: A study of the prevalence of abuse and neglect.* www.nspcc.org.uk/inform

Clemmons, J. C., Walsh, K., DiLillo, D., & Messman-Moore, T. L. (2007). Unique and combined contributions of multiple child abuse types and abuse severity to adult trauma symptomatology. *Child Maltreatment, 12*(2), 172–181. https://doi.org/10.1177/1077559506298248

Collishaw, S., Pickles, A., Messer, J., Rutter, M., Shearer, C., & Maughan, B. (2007). Resilience to adult psychopathology following childhood maltreatment: Evidence from a community sample. *Child Abuse & Neglect, 31*(3), 211–229. https://doi.org/10.1016/j.chiabu.2007.02.004

Courtois, C. A., & Courtois Riley, C. (1992). Pregnancy and childbirth as triggers for abuse memories: Implications for care. *Birth, 19*(4), 222–223.

De Paúl, J., & Domenech, L. (2000). Childhood history of abuse and child abuse potential in adolescent mothers: A longitudinal study. *Child Abuse & Neglect, 24*(5), 701–713. https://doi.org/10.1016/s0145-2134(00)00124-1

Donaldson, P. E., Whalen, M. H., & Anastas, J. W. (1989). Teen pregnancy and sexual abuse: Exploring the connection. *Smith College Studies in Social Work, 59*(3), 289–300. https://doi.org/10.1080/00377318909517360

Dong, M., Anda, R. F., Felitti, V. J., Dube, S. R., Williamson, D. F., Thompson, T. J., Loo, C. M., & Giles, W. H. (2004). The interrelatedness of multiple forms of childhood abuse, neglect, and household dysfunction. *Child Abuse & Neglect, 28*(7), 771–784. https://doi.org/10.1016/j.chiabu.2004.01.008

Felitti, V. J. M. D., Anda, R. F. M. D., Nordenberg, D. M. D., Williamson, D. F. M. S., Spitz, A. M. M. S., Edwards, V. B. A., Koss, M. P. P., & Marks, J. S. M. D. (1998). Relationship of childhood abuse and household dysfunction to many of the leading causes of death in adults: The Adverse Childhood Experiences (ACE) Study. *American Journal of Preventive Medicine, 14*(4), 245–258. https://doi.org/10.1016/S0749-3797(98)00017-8

Ferguson, K. S., & Dacey, C. M. (1997). Anxiety, depression, and dissociation in women health care providers reporting a history of childhood psychological abuse. *Child Abuse & Neglect, 21*(10), 941–952. https://doi.org/10.1016/S0145-2134(97)00055-0

Finkelhor, D. (1979). *Sexually victimized children*. Collier Macmillan Publishers.

Finkelhor, D. (1994). Current information on the scope and nature of child sexual abuse. *The Future of Children, 4*, 31–53.

Finkelhor, D., Ormrod, R. K., & Turner, H. A. (2007). Poly-victimization: A neglected component in child victimization. *Child Abuse & Neglect, 31*(1), 7–26. https://doi.org/10.1016/j.chiabu.2006.06.008

Ford, D. C., Merrick, M. T., Parks, S. E., Breiding, M. J., Gilbert, L. K., Edwards, V. J., Dhingra, S. S., Barile, J. P., & Thompson, W. W. (2014). Examination of the factorial structure of adverse childhood experiences and recommendations for three subscale scores. *Psychology of Violence, 4*(4), 432–444. https://doi.org/10.1037/a0037723

Garbarino, J. (1989). The psychologically battered child: Toward a definition. *Pediatric Annals, 18*(8), 502–504.

Garbarino, J. (2013). The emotionally battered child. In R. D. Krugman & J. E. Korbin (Eds.), *C. Henry Kempe: A 50 year legacy to the field of child abuse and neglect* (pp. 57–61). Springer.

Gelaye, B., Kajeepeta, S., Zhong, Q.-Y., Borba, C. P., Rondon, M. B., Sánchez, S. E., Henderson, D. C., & Williams, M. A. (2015). Childhood abuse is associated with stress-related sleep disturbance and poor sleep quality in pregnancy. *Sleep Medicine, 16*(10), 1274–1280. https://doi.org/10.1016/j.sleep.2015.07.004

Giallo, R., Pilkington, P., McDonald, E., Gartland, D., Woolhouse, H., & Brown, S. (2017). Physical, sexual and social health factors associated with the trajectories of maternal depressive symptoms from pregnancy to 4 years postpartum. *Social Psychiatry and Psychiatric Epidemiology, 52*(7), 815–828. https://doi.org/10.1007/s00127-017-1387-8

Grimstad, H., & Schei, B. (1999). Pregnancy and delivery for women with a history of child sexual abuse. *Child Abuse & Neglect, 23*(1), 81–90. https://doi.org/10.1016/s0145-2134(98)00113-6

Haugaard, J. J. (2000). The challenge of defining child sexual abuse. *American Psychologist, 55*(9), 1036–1039. https://doi.org/10.1037//0003-066X.55.9.1036

Heimstad, R., Dahloe, R., Laache, I., Skogvoll, E., & Schei, B. (2006). Fear of childbirth and history of abuse: Implications for pregnancy and delivery. *Acta Obstetricia et Gynecologica Scandinavica, 85*(4), 435–440. https://doi.org/10.1080/00016340500432507

Higgins, D. J., & McCabe, M. P. (2001). Multiple forms of child abuse and neglect: Adult retrospective reports. *Aggression and Violent Behavior, 6*(6), 547–578. https://doi.org/10.1016/S1359-1789(00)00030-6

Hulme, P. A. (2004). Retrospective measurement of childhood sexual abuse: A review of instruments. *Child Maltreatment, 9*(2), 201–217. https://doi.org/10.1177/1077559504264264

IPSCAN. (2008). *World perspectives on child abuse.* https://cwrp.ca/sites/default/files/publications/en/ISPCAN_World_Perspectives_Child_Abuse_2008.pdf

Issokson, D. (2004). *Effects of childhood abuse on childbearing and perinatal health.* American Psychological Association.

Kempe, C. H., Silverman, F. N., Steele, B. F., Droegemueller, W., & Silver, H. K. (1985). The battered-child syndrome. *Child Abuse & Neglect, 9,* 143–154. https://doi.org/10.1016/0145-2134(85)90005-5

Lacey, R. E., & Minnis, H. (2020). Practitioner Review: Twenty years of research with adverse childhood experience scores - Advantages, disadvantages and applications to practice. *Journal of Child Psychology and Psychiatry, 61*(2), 116–130. https://doi.org/10.1111/jcpp.13135

Lang, A. J., Gartstein, M. A., Rodgers, C. S., & Lebeck, M. M. (2010). The impact of maternal childhood abuse on parenting and infant temperament. *Journal of Child Adolescent Psychiatric Nursing, 23*(2), 100–110. https://doi. org/10.1111/j.1744-6171.2010.00229.x

Lanier, P., Maguire-Jack, K., Lombardi, B., Frey, J., & Rose, R. A. (2018). Adverse childhood experiences and child health outcomes: Comparing cumulative risk and latent class approaches. *Maternal and Child Health Journal, 22*(3), 288–297. https://doi.org/10.1007/s10995-017-2365-1

Leeb, R. T., Lewis, T., & Zolotor, A. J. (2011). A review of physical and mental health consequences of child abuse and neglect and implications for practice. *American Journal of Lifestyle Medicine, 5*(5), 454–468. https://doi. org/10.1177/1559827611410266

Leeb, R. T., Paulozzi, L., Melanson, C., Simon, T., & Aria, I. (2008). Child maltreatment surveillance: Uniform definitions for public health and recommended data elements, Version 1.0. http://www.cdc.gov/ncipc/dvp/CMP/CMP-Surveillance.htm

Leeners, B., Gorres, G., Block, E., & Hengartner, M. P. (2016). Birth experiences in adult women with a history of childhood sexual abuse. *Journal of Psychosomatic Research, 83*, 27–32. https://doi.org/10.1016/j.jpsychores.2016.02.006

Leeners, B., Stiller, R., Block, E., Görres, G., Imthurn, B., & Rath, W. (2007). Effect of childhood sexual abuse on gynecologic care as an adult. *Psychosomatics, 48*(5), 385–393. https://doi.org/10.1176/appi.psy.48.5.385

LoCascio, M., Infurna, M. R., Guarnaccia, C., Mancuso, L., Bifulco, A., & Giannone, F. (2018). Does childhood psychological abuse contribute to intimate partner violence victimization? An investigation using the childhood experience of care and abuse interview. *Journal of Interpersonal Violence, 36*, NP4626. https://doi.org/10.1177/0886260518794512

Logan, C., Holcombe, E., Ryan, S., Manlove, J., & Moore, K. (2007). *Childhood sexual abuse and teen pregnancy*. https://dpi.wi.gov/sites/default/files/imce/sspw/pdf/inspireabuseandpreg_2007.pdf

Lukasse, M., Vangen, S., Oian, P., Kumle, M., Ryding, E. L., & Schei, B. (2010). Childhood abuse and fear of childbirth—A population-based study. *Birth: Issues in Perinatal Care, 37*(4), 267–274. https://doi. org/10.1111/j.1523-536X.2010.00420.x

Mathews, B., Pacella, R., Dunne, M., Scott, J., Finkelhor, D., Meinck, F., Higgins, D. J., Erskine, H., Thomas, H. J., Haslam, D., Tran, N., Le, H., Honey, N., Kellard, K., & Lawrence, D. (2021). The Australian Child Maltreatment Study (ACMS): Protocol for a national survey of the prevalence of child abuse and neglect, associated mental disorders and physical health problems, and burden of disease. *BMJ Open, 11*(5), e047074. https:// doi.org/10.1136/bmjopen-2020-047074

Mathews, B. P., Walsh, K. M., Dunne, M. P., Katz, I., Arney, F., Higgins, D., Octoman, O., Parkinson, S., & Bates, S. (2016). *Scoping study for research into the prevalence of child abuse in Australia: Final report.* Prepared for the Royal Commission into Institutional Responses to Child Sexual Abuse. https://eprints.qut.edu.au/103910/

Matsumoto, M., Piersiak, H. A., Letterie, M. C., & Humphreys, K. L. (2020). Population-based estimates of associations between child maltreatment types: A meta-analysis. *Trauma, Violence, & Abuse., 24,* 487. https://doi. org/10.1177/15248380211030502

Melender, H.-L. (2002). Fears and coping strategies associated with pregnancy and childbirth in Finland. *Journal of Midwifery & Women's Health, 47*(4), 256–263. https://doi.org/10.1016/S1526-9523(02)00263-5

Moody, G., Cannings-John, R., Hood, K., Kemp, A., & Robling, M. (2018). Establishing the international prevalence of self-reported child maltreatment: A systematic review by maltreatment type and gender. *BMC Public Health, 18*(1), 1164. https://doi.org/10.1186/s12889-018-6044-y

Newberger, E. H., Zuidema, G. D., & Nardi, G. L. (Eds.). (1982). *Child abuse.* Little Brown and Company.

Nidey, N., Bowers, K., Ammerman, R. T., Shah, A. N., Phelan, K. J., Clark, M. J., Van Ginkel, J. B., & Folger, A. T. (2020). Combinations of adverse childhood events and risk of postpartum depression among mothers enrolled in a home visiting program. *Annals of Epidemiology, 52,* 26–34. https://doi. org/10.1016/j.annepidem.2020.09.015

O'Hagan, K. P. (1993). *Emotional and psychological abuse of children.* Open University Press.

O'Hagan, K. P. (1995). Emotional and psychological abuse: Problems of definition. *Child Abuse & Neglect, 19*(4), 449–461. https://doi. org/10.1016/0145-2134(95)00006-T

Ornduff, S. R., Kelsey, R. M., Bursi, C., Alpert, B. S., & Bada, H. S. (2002). Child abuse potential in at-risk African American mothers: The role of life experience variables. *American Journal of Orthopsychiatry, 72*(3), 433–444. https://doi.org/10.1037/0002-9432.72.3.433

Price-Robertson, R., Higgins, D. J., & Vassallo, S. (2013). *Multi-type maltreatment and polyvictimisation. A comparison of two frameworks.* https://aifs.gov. au/research/family-matters/no-93/multi-type-maltreatment-and-polyvictimisation.

Putnam, F. W. (2003). Ten-year research update Review: Child sexual abuse. *Journal of the American Academy of Child & Adolescent Psychiatry, 42*(3), 269–278. https://doi.org/10.1097/00004583-200303000-00006

Qiao, D., & Chan, Y.-C. (2005). Child abuse in China: A yet-to-be-acknowledged 'social problem' in the Chinese mainland. *Child & Family Social Work, 10*(1), 21–27. https://doi.org/10.1111/j.1365-2206.2005.00347.x

Radford, L., Corral, S., Bradley, C., Fisher, H., Bassett, C., Howat, N., & Collishaw, S. (2011). *Child abuse and neglect in the UK today*. https://learning.nspcc.org.uk/research-resources/pre-2013/child-abuse-neglect-uk-today.

Rhodes, N., & Hutchinson, S. (1994). Labor experiences of childhood sexual abuse survivors. *Birth, 21*(4), 213–220. https://doi.org/10.1111/j.1523-536X.1994.tb00532.x

Robinson, Y. (2019). Child abuse: Types and emergent issues. In I. Bryce, Y. Robinson, & W. Petherick (Eds.), *Child abuse and neglect. Forensic issues in evidence, impact, and management*. Academic Press.

Rose, A. (1992). Effects of childhood sexual abuse on childbirth: One Woman's story. *Birth, 19*(4), 214–218. https://doi.org/10.1111/j.1523-536X.1992.tb00405.x

Russell, D. E. H. (1984). *Sexual exploitation: Rape, child sexual abuse, and workplace harassment*. SAGE Publications.

Selk, S. C., Rich-Edwards, J. W., Koenen, K., & Kubzansky, L. D. (2016). An observational study of type, timing, and severity of childhood maltreatment and preterm birth. *Journal of Epidemiology and Community Health, 70*(6), 589–595. https://doi.org/10.1136/jech-2015-206304

Solomon, T. (1973). History and demography of child abuse. *Pediatrics, 51*(4), 773–776.

Souch, A. J., Jones, I. R., Shelton, K. H. M., & Waters, C. S. (2022). Maternal childhood maltreatment and perinatal outcomes: A systematic review. *Journal of Affective Disorders, 302*, 139–159. https://doi.org/10.1016/j.jad.2022.01.062

Stoltenborgh, M., Bakermans-Kranenburg, M. J., Alink, L. R., & van IJzendoorn, M. H. (2015). The prevalence of child maltreatment across the globe: Review of a series of meta-analyses. *Child Abuse Review, 24*(1), 37–50. https://doi.org/10.1002/car.2353

Strathearn, L., Giannotti, M., Mills, R., Kisely, S., Najman, J., & Abajobir, A. (2020). Long-term cognitive, psychological, and health outcomes associated with child abuse and neglect. *Pediatrics, 146*(4). https://doi.org/10.1542/peds.2020-0438

The World Counts. (2022). *World population*. https://www.theworldcounts.com

WHO. (1999). *World Health Organization. 1999. Report of the consultation on child abuse prevention 29–31 March 1999.* https://apps.who.int/iris/handle/10665/65900

World Population Review. (2022). *Age of consent by country 2022.* https://worldpopulationreview.com/country-rankings/age-of-consent-by-country

Zhang, X., Sun, J., Wang, J., Chen, Q., Cao, D., Wang, J., & Cao, F. (2020). Suicide ideation among pregnant women: The role of different experiences of childhood abuse. *Journal of Affective Disorders, 266,* 182–186. https://doi.org/10.1016/j.jad.2020.01.119

3

Theoretical Perspectives of Child Abuse

Robyn Brunton ⓘ and Rachel Dryer ⓘ

Abstract This chapter provides an overview of six theories that describe and explain child abuse and its potential sequelae for perinatal women. Theories examined include cascade models that provide a framework for understanding the progressive effects of adversity. Differential susceptibility theory highlights the individual characteristics that increase or reduce an individual's vulnerability to adversity. Experiential avoidance seeks to explain behaviors used to cope with distress (e.g., substance use, self-harm) and how disassociation can be a means of coping with distressing childbirth. Resilience theories provide insights into the opportunities for positive interventions. The traumagenic dynamics model was initially developed for child sexual abuse but has the potential for broader

R. Brunton (✉)
School of Psychology, Charles Sturt University, Bathurst, NSW, Australia
e-mail: rbrunton@csu.edu.au

R. Dryer
School of Behavioural & Health Sciences (Faculty of Health Science),
Australian Catholic University, Strathfield, NSW, Australia
e-mail: rachel.dryer@acu.edu.au

application in demonstrating the sequelae of abuse. Finally, while limited in its application for perinatal research, the stress sensitization model can explain some psychological outcomes related to abuse and perinatal women. The theories and models reviewed in this chapter account for the transactional nature of the individual experiences of childhood abuse and have explanatory power for perinatal research.

Keywords Cascade models • Differential susceptibility • Experiential avoidance • Resilience • Traumagenic • Stress sensitization

Theories explain the cause and effect of phenomena and provide a unifying framework for understanding a psychological construct or phenomenon, the behaviors associated with that construct or phenomenon, and the factors that contribute to or influence development. By drawing on the topics of this book, this chapter provides an overview of six theories that provide descriptions and explanations of research findings on child abuse and its potential sequelae or positive adaptation and functioning for perinatal women.

Developmental Cascade Theories

Developmental cascade models[1] provide a theoretical framework to understand the influence of early life adversity on cognitive, social, and emotional developmental outcomes. These models explain the influence on human development of interactions and transactions of various effects that can promote or hinder development. Cascade effects can be direct, indirect, unidirectional, or bidirectional, all potentially altering the course of development (Masten & Cicchetti, 2010).

Cascade effects are also cumulative, with each developmental event building on the previous event, gaining momentum, and contributing to subsequent cascades in a dose-response manner (Giovanelli et al., 2020).

---

[1] Also known as chain reactions, snowballs, amplification, spillover, progressive, and cumulative effects (Giovanelli et al., 2020; Masten & Cicchetti, 2010).

For example, early adversity can contribute to health risk behaviors before and during pregnancy and postpartum, leading to poorer outcomes for the mother and her child (see Fig. 3.1).

As shown above, the impact of child abuse can snowball over the life course, interacting with the individual's larger sociocultural context. Moreover, cascade models explain why some women who experience multiple adversities have worse outcomes than those with fewer instances of adversity. For example, a history of child abuse is a risk factor for postpartum depression; however, experiencing both child abuse and intimate partner violence during pregnancy doubles this risk (Mahenge et al., 2018).

Cascade models have been examined with respect to intergenerational outcomes. For example, using sequential mediation, Russotti et al. (2020) examined the maternal history of child maltreatment (physical, sexual, psychological abuse, or neglect), identifying multigenerational developmental effects. They found that maternal maltreatment predicted chronic offspring maltreatment, which, in turn, predicted higher externalizing symptoms for the child (e.g., conduct problems, behavior). They also identified that maltreatment predicted maternal depression leading to greater offspring internalizing symptoms (e.g., child depression, anxiety, poor emotional functioning). Finally, they noted that children born to

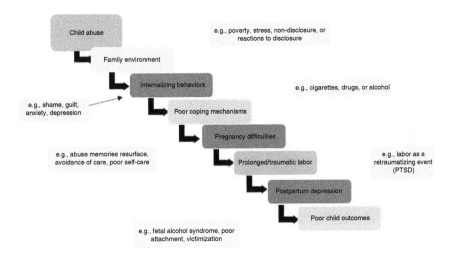

Fig. 3.1 Conceptualizing the cascading effects of child abuse

mothers who began childbearing during adolescence were more likely to experience chronic child maltreatment and develop subsequent externalizing symptoms. Other recent studies further support developmental cascades. These include Coe et al. (2021), who found that only women who reported high maternal adverse childhood experiences were associated with maternal intimate partner violence and depressive symptoms. Additionally, Russotti et al. (2020) identified in a prospective, longitudinal study that adolescent pregnancy amplified the effect of maternal experiences of child maltreatment on depressive symptoms during late adolescence.

Differential Susceptibility Theory

Differential susceptibility theory provides a lens to explain why some children are more susceptible to the adverse effects of risky environments and the beneficial effects of supportive environments. This theory builds on previous diathesis-stress or transactional/dual risk models by proposing that natural selection provides development processes that vary a child's susceptibility to environmental and other influences of child rearing. This variation protects children from being steered in a single developmental direction that may be unfavorable in the future (Belsky, 2013; Boyce & Ellis, 2005). Therefore, according to this theory, adverse experiences do not disrupt development but rather "direct or regulate" it toward adaptive strategies that may seem harmful in the long-term but are necessary to ensure survival (Ellis et al., 2011, p. 8). For example, parental neglect may enhance learned fearful and defensive behaviors in a child, accelerate their sexual maturation, and also lessen parental investment in the offspring (Ellis et al., 2011). While these may appear unfavorable, they promote the child's survival. An important aspect of this perspective is that some individuals with a disproportionate vulnerability to risk-promoting environments (e.g., maltreatment) may also get a disproportionate benefit from favorable environments (e.g., supportive, secure). As a result, they are more reactive to these different environments than other children.[2]

This differential susceptibility to the environment may come from genes that moderate or interact with environmental exposures on developmental outcomes. Therefore, individuals may differ in their neurobiological susceptibility to the environment. Put simply, individuals may inherit certain traits or vulnerabilities that mediate or moderate their susceptibility to adversity. Research into gene and environment (GxE) interactions and polygenetic plasticity (GxG) support this model (see Belsky, 2013 for an overview). For example, research has identified that a particular variant of the DRD4 dopamine receptor gene moderates the relationship between unresolved maternal loss or trauma and infant attachment disorganization (Bakermans-Kranenburg & Van Ijzendoorn, 2011).

From a developmental psychology viewpoint, this differential susceptibility operates across the life span, and not just in a single developmental period. Changes are sustained through adaptation, but this does not preclude the possibility of transient changes. In addition, the heightened neurobiological susceptibility increases the likelihood that good outcomes will come from positive environments (e.g., secure attachment, high self-esteem), and poorer outcomes from more negative environments (e.g., substance abuse, depression). Figure 3.2 shows a conceptual overview of the theory.

This theory highlights limitations in extant research by demonstrating that individual characteristics may moderate differential outcomes, not just contextual effects. Therefore, when researchers only examine the effect of child abuse on a particular outcome that applies equally to all children (i.e., the main effect), without considering any interaction between the environment and individuals, their findings are limited (Belsky, 2013).

Concerning the literature on perinatal child abuse survivors, several studies have examined potential individual and biological influences on the relationship between adversity and outcome. For example, Van

---

[2] Ellis et al. (2011) called these children orchid children (more susceptible to different environments) and dandelion children (ability to function across different environments).

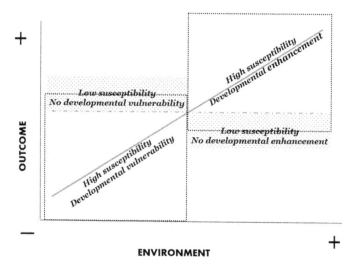

Fig. 3.2 A conceptual overview of differential susceptibility theory (adapted from Ellis et al., 2011)

Ijzendoorn and Bakermans-Kranenburg (2006) identified DRD4 7-repeat, a dopamine-related gene, as increasing the risk for disorganization in children raised by mothers with unresolved loss or trauma (death of a relative). However, children with DRD4 7-repeat raised by mothers with no loss or trauma had less disorganization than children without this gene, regardless of the mother's loss or trauma status. Furthermore, replicating these findings with other dopamine-related genes (see systematic review and meta-analysis by Bakermans-Kranenburg & Van Ijzendoorn, 2011) demonstrates that characterizing these genes as vulnerabilities is a misnomer given their differential functioning.

Experiential Avoidance

Research studies have demonstrated that survivors of child abuse have a higher likelihood of substance use (i.e., cigarettes, alcohol, and drugs) during pregnancy and postpartum than women who have not had these experiences (for a review, see Brunton, 2022). While there are limited studies in this area, there are indications that pregnant women who experienced child abuse are more likely to smoke or consume alcohol than women with low or no trauma experiences (Blalock et al., 2011; Cammack, 2017; Racine et al., 2020). In studies that have examined drug use during pregnancy, women reporting a history of child sexual or physical abuse were more likely to use illicit drugs (Jantzen et al., 1998). This greater substance use has been partly attributed to child abuse survivors employing avoidant coping strategies to numb or avoid associated negative emotions (Arslan, 2017).

There is no unified theory of experiential avoidance. Instead, several theories recognize that experiential avoidance[3] is a process with the underlying proposition that a person is seeking to escape the consequences of an adverse experience (Hayes et al., 1996). Experiential avoidance includes escape and avoidance in any form, and substance abuse can be a means of numbing or forgetting victimization experiences, memories, or related affective responses (Chawla & Ostafin, 2007). This escapism, when in the form of antenatal substance use, can be costly to the developing fetus as it introduces harmful teratogens into the prenatal environment. Zero-tolerance approaches by governments and policymakers (e.g., CDC, 2021) recognize these potential and harmful consequences, such as congenital disabilities and malformation and the potential for developmental disorders (e.g., fetal alcohol spectrum disorders, Keegan et al., 2010).

Resilience Theories

Resilience theories have wide application in many fields (e.g., psychology, sociology, social work), applying to individuals, families, communities, and workplaces with a focus on strengths that enable people to rise above adversity (van Breda, 2018). The emergence of these theories was consistent with a move from deficit models that examine pathogenesis (origins of disease) to strengths-based models that examine salutogenesis (origins of health) (van Breda, 2018).

---

[3] Also known as emotional or cognitive avoidance (Hayes et al., 1996).

Resilience can be understood as how children overcome adversity to achieve good developmental outcomes or positive adaptation; some children flourish amid adversity (Masten & Coatsworth, 1998). This approach acknowledges that resilience is a process[4] that provides a capacity to recover from or adapt to adversity. Therefore, consistent with this view, resilience mediates between adversity and positive outcomes (see Fig. 3.3).

Resilience theories focus on the protective processes against risks that may disrupt or hinder positive development. While there is no single unifying theory, the underlying premise of resilience theories is that resilience emerges from complex interactions between multilevel systems of functioning (e.g., individual, family, environment) in a person's life. These include gene-environment correlations (e.g., systematic interrelationships between the two) or gene-environment interactions (e.g., the interplay between genes and environment) and highlight the role of developmental timing on the development and manifestation of resilience.

With respect to resilience theories, outcomes can be chronic (i.e., extended period) or acute (i.e., briefer duration with a clear starting point, van Breda, 2018). Chronic outcomes can be further classified as having a distal or proximal onset. Distal onset adversity has no starting

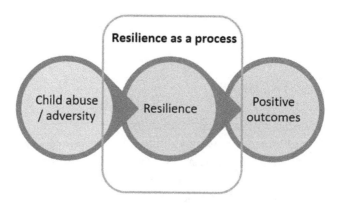

Fig. 3.3 Resilience as a process (adapted from van Breda, 2018)

---

[4] Some researchers make the distinction of resilience as an outcome; see van Breda (2018) for a fuller discussion.

point for an individual, such as abuse that extends from birth or early infancy. Proximal, however, has an apparent onset. These differences are essential in recognizing the different pathways of resilience. Acute and proximal chronic adversities may allow a person to return to pre-adversity levels. Conversely, distal onset (chronic) with no pre-abuse levels means the individual may develop sustained coping or stress resistance.

Much research has focused on intra-personal and interpersonal factors as resilience processes. These factors include hardiness, self-efficacy, intelligence, attachment, and peer relationships (Masten, 2007; van Breda, 2018). However, in the perinatal literature, mediators that are often considered are risk-promoting (see Appleyard et al., 2011; Choi, 2018), consistent with a deficit-based approach. Nevertheless, resilience-based models can help expand our understanding of the gene-environment interplay on development that promotes good outcomes. Only a few studies have examined resilience in perinatal women (e.g., Brunton et al., 2020; Chung et al., 2008), with these studies identifying that resilience factors (e.g., positive relationships), or resilience in general (i.e., ability to bounce back or recover), mediate the relationship between maternal experiences of child abuse and poor outcomes.

Traumagenic Dynamics Model (Finkelhor & Browne, 1985)

Traumagenic dynamics are trauma-causing factors that mediate the outcomes of child sexual abuse. This model proposes four traumagenic dynamics: traumatic sexualization, betrayal, stigmatization, and powerlessness. Traumatic sexualization occurs because child sexual abuse is developmentally inappropriate and interpersonally dysfunctional. This abuse can result in inappropriate learning, such as misconceptions about sexual behavior and morality. This aspect of trauma can also mean that traumatic memories of abuse reemerge as they are associated with sexuality. Feelings of betrayal can come from losing a trusted person who perpetrates the abuse, others who are unwilling or unable to offer protection, or those who disbelieve or ostracize when the abuse is disclosed to them.

Stigmatization results from the negative connotations of child abuse communicated to the child, which can be explicit such as pressures to maintain secrecy, demeaning behavior, or being blamed for the abuse. These messages can also be implicit through social attitudes reinforcing that child abuse is deviant or taboo. Negative connotations are further strengthened if their disclosure is met with shock, hysteria, or blame. Finally, a child feels powerlessness as the abuse contravenes their will, leading to distortions of their sense of control and self-efficacy. Disempowerment can also come from the failure to stop the abuse, either through their efforts or by seeking help which reinforces their dependency on others (because they are a child).

Only a few studies have examined this model, providing some empirical support (e.g., Cantón-Cortés et al., 2012; Kallstrom-Fuqua et al., 2004). Notwithstanding this, the model, derived from findings within the literature, provides an organizing framework for outcomes associated with perinatal survivors of child abuse. For instance, the previous traumatic sexualization of child sexual abuse survivors explains why they have a greater likelihood of high-risk sexual behaviors, such as earlier sexual activity or less effective birth control (Noll et al., 2003). These risky behaviors can lead to an adolescent, teenage, or unplanned pregnancy (Dietz et al., 1999; Drevin, 2019; Garwood et al., 2015; Noll et al., 2003). Traumatic sexualization also explains why child sexual abuse survivors have a greater fear of childbirth and associated intimate procedures, and experience flashbacks of the abuse during gynecological consultations, childbirth, or pregnancy in general, commonly associated with invasive or unexpected examinations (Leeners et al., 2016; Leeners et al., 2007; Leeners et al., 2013; Lukasse et al., 2010). These procedures involve body parts typically associated with sexual activity (Leeners et al., 2006), which could trigger these aversive reactions. These flashbacks, sometimes, are the first reemergence of abuse memories since their occurrence (Leeners et al., 2016). Finally, traumatic sexualization can impair judgment about people's trustworthiness or vulnerability to unhealthy relationships. This explains why child sexual abuse survivors have an increased risk of revictimization during pregnancy or throughout their lifetime (Barnett et al., 2018; Barrios et al., 2015).

With respect to stigmatization, Finkelhor and Browne (1985) propose that it can lead to feelings of guilt or shame, isolation, and involvement in drugs, alcohol, or prostitution. In extreme cases, they propose that stigmatization can result in self-destructive and self-harming behaviors or suicide. Consistent with this proposition, survivors of child sexual abuse have higher distress or depression (Chung et al., 2008; Yampolsky et al., 2010) and are more likely to smoke and consume alcohol (Blalock et al., 2011; Racine et al., 2020) during pregnancy and postpartum than non-abused women. There are also indications that child physical and sexual abuse are risk factors for suicide ideation (Zhang et al., 2020).

The traumagenic dynamic of betrayal can manifest as distrust of other people, which explains why some child abuse survivors have more difficulty with relationships during pregnancy and postpartum. For instance, abuse survivors may avoid birth preparation classes (as the experience of lying down among strangers is frightening) and have difficulty trusting healthcare providers (Leeners et al., 2013). All these factors can impact their prenatal care.

Powerlessness relates to several interrelated effects, such as fear and anxiety, nightmares, and somatic complaints. This dynamic explains why some abuse survivors have increased fears for their unborn baby's welfare (as they perceive the world as unsafe, Chamberlain et al., 2019; Eide et al., 2010) and more pregnancy-related anxiety overall (Brunton et al., 2020), and more significant somatic complaints during pregnancy (Littleton, 2015; Lukasse et al., 2009). Powerlessness is also related to a lower sense of self-efficacy, consistent with child abuse survivors (physical and sexual abuse) scoring lower on measures of parenting self-efficacy when dealing with a difficult infant (Kunseler et al., 2016).

An integral aspect of this model is that the traumagenic dynamics do not apply solely to the abuse event. For example, previous experiences, such as family instability and poor family relationships, may have already disempowered the child. Conversely, an older child may have a well-developed self-concept and self-efficacy and feel powerful through healthy family roles. These can be risk factors, or they may protect and dilute the disempowering aspects of any subsequent abuse. Events after the abuse could also impact the traumagenic dynamics, such as disclosing the abuse and reactions to this disclosure. Finkelhor and Browne (1985) identified the family's reaction and social and institutional responses as two main aspects of disclosure. In either category, disclosure could be positive or negative. For instance, any stigma around the abuse experience (discussed above) may elicit adverse reactions. In contrast, if a child is supported and protected post-disclosure, this may mitigate any sense of powerlessness from the sexual abuse.

Given these considerations, the model highlights the importance of moderating and mediating effects. Brunton et al. (2020) identified resilience and social support as moderators of maternal child abuse experience and pregnancy-related anxiety, which can be linked to these pre- and post-factors. However, few studies have examined environmental, societal, and institutional influences on perinatal outcomes, which are worthy of further exploration.

The Stress Sensitization Model

The stress sensitization model was first proposed to explain the association between psychosocial stressors and affective disorders (Post, 1992). The model posits that those who have suffered early stressors such as maltreatment become sensitized to stress through memory-like mechanisms and are more vulnerable to further psychopathology. Underlying this sensitization (i.e., increased reactivity to future stressors) are neurobiological processes. Furthermore, these processes can have longer-term effects by altering gene expression, that is, epigenetic effects.[5]

In 1992, Post postulated that neurobiological changes from repeated stress result in progressive behavioral and physiological increases in reactivity. Therefore, the first affective disorder episode would likely be preceded by major psychological stressors than subsequent episodes. After initial sensitization to stressors, reoccurrences of psychopathology can increasingly occur independently of such events (i.e., major psychological stressors). Furthermore, continued stress can increase responsivity to

---

[5] Epigenetic effects are ways in which environmental influences alter the expression of genes (whether they are turned on or off).

psychopathology; therefore, successive stressors can elicit stronger affective and behavioral responses over time (Stroud et al., 2020).

This model was originally formulated to explain affective disorders but expanded to acknowledge that early adversity can lead to epigenetic modifications that increase sensitivity to later stress and a broader range of psychopathology (e.g., post-traumatic stress disorder [PTSD], anxiety disorders, obsessive compulsive disorder) (Post, 2016). Concerning perinatal women, this stressor could be childbirth, with research supporting that for some women, childbirth can trigger PTSD symptomology (Lev-Wiesel & Daphna-Tekoah, 2010).

The model has good empirical support, with later epigenetic research supporting Post's early theorizing (Post, 2016). Notwithstanding this, limitations in extant research support the need for further research (see Stroud et al., 2020, for a review). With respect to the perinatal literature, the model provides a lens to understand the identified links between early childhood adversity and affective disorders. For example, Hutchens et al. (2017) conducted an integrative review (six cross-sectional and 10 longitudinal studies), identifying consistent associations between child maltreatment and postpartum depression. The strongest effect was for a study on maternal childhood physical abuse, which increased the odds of postpartum depression by 5.5 times (Plaza et al., 2012). Also, consistent with the model, Records and Rice (2009) identified that women with a history of lifetime abuse were nearly four times more likely to have depression four months postpartum and eight times more likely at eight months postpartum.

Conclusion

The theories and models reviewed in this chapter all account for the transactional nature of individual experiences and their environment and have explanatory power for perinatal research on maternal experiences of child abuse. Despite no single unifying theory, cascade models provide a framework for understanding the progressive effects of adversity. For some children, the cumulating consequences of child abuse (e.g., poverty, familial influences) that occur via multiple processes and pathways can snowball over time. Importantly, however, these models acknowledge the bidirectional nature of cascade effects providing a theoretical understanding of both positive and negative influences. However, examining these influences and effects requires comprehensive longitudinal designs that can be costly and time-consuming. Differential susceptibility theory highlights that individual characteristics may increase or reduce an individual's vulnerability to adversity. However, research within the perinatal literature has historically focused on risk-promoting factors rather than development-enhancing environmental conditions. Research such as that conducted by Van Ijzendoorn and Bakermans-Kranenburg (2006) provides a deeper understanding of adversity's impacts and potential resilience or vulnerability factors.

While experiential avoidance generally explains substance use as a means of coping, avoidance can take other forms, such as obsessive-compulsive behaviors to reduce or avoid anxiety and self-harming (e.g., cutting or suicide) to reduce or avoid distressing feelings. Moreover, disassociation during childbirth could be a means of avoidance for abuse sufferers with PTSD (Leeners et al., 2016). Also, avoiding close interpersonal relationships is another coping method that affects care and support (Hayes et al., 1996). Therefore, experimental avoidance has the potential for broader application within child abuse research. Resilience theories demonstrate that examining different resilience factors enables insights into opportunities during pregnancy and postpartum to circumvent poor outcomes. The traumagenic dynamics model demonstrates the sequelae of these poor outcomes. Research supports the link between child sexual abuse and these dynamics, as shown in the perinatal literature. While this model initially focused on child sexual abuse, this does not preclude other abuses (e.g., physical, emotional, psychological) from having the same outcomes. Indeed, many studies cited above showed similar effects for other abuse types. However, the conjunction of these dynamics makes them unique to sexual abuse (Finkelhor & Browne, 1985). Finally, the stress sensitization model has good explanatory power for some psychological outcomes but is limited in its application for perinatal research. For example, outcomes related to intergenerational effects, somatic symptoms, and differential outcomes fall outside the scope of this model. Moreover, while the stress sensitization model has generated interventions for clinical application, its deficit-based approach limits its explanatory power.

References

Appleyard, K., Berlin, L., Rosanbalm, K., & Dodge, K. (2011). Preventing early child maltreatment: Implications from a longitudinal study of maternal abuse history, substance use problems, and offspring victimization. *Prevention Science, 12*(2), 139–149. https://doi.org/10.1007/s11121-010-0193-2

Arslan, G. (2017). Psychological maltreatment, coping strategies, and mental health problems: A brief and effective measure of psychological maltreatment in adolescents. *Child Abuse & Neglect, 68*, 96–106. https://doi.org/10.1016/j.chiabu.2017.03.023

Bakermans-Kranenburg, M. J., & Van Ijzendoorn, M. H. (2011). Differential susceptibility to rearing environment depending on dopamine-related genes: New evidence and a meta-analysis. *Development and Psychopathology, 23*(1), 39–52. https://doi.org/10.1017/S0954579410000635

Barnett, W., Halligan, S., Heron, J., Fraser, A., Koen, N., Zar, H. J., Donald, K. A., & Stein, D. J. (2018). Maltreatment in childhood and intimate partner violence: A latent class growth analysis in a South African pregnancy cohort. *Child Abuse & Neglect, 86*, 336–348. https://doi.org/10.1016/j.chiabu.2018.08.020

Barrios, Y. V., Gelaye, B., Zhong, Q., Nicolaidis, C., Rondon, M. B., Garcia, P. J., Sanchez, P. A., Sanchez, S. E., & Williams, M. A. (2015). Association of childhood physical and sexual abuse with intimate partner violence, poor general health and depressive symptoms among pregnant women. *PLoS One, 10*(1), e0116609. https://doi.org/10.1371/journal.pone.0116609

Belsky, J. (2013). Differential susceptibility to environmental influences. *International Journal of Child Care and Education Policy, 7*(2), 15–31. https://doi.org/10.1007/2288-6729-7-2-15

Blalock, J. A., Nayak, N., Wetter, D. W., Schreindorfer, L., Minnix, J. A., Canul, J., & Cinciripini, P. M. (2011). The relationship of childhood trauma to nicotine dependence in pregnant smokers. *Psychology of Addictive Behaviors, 25*(4), 652–663. https://doi.org/10.1037/a0025529

Boyce, W. T., & Ellis, B. J. (2005). Biological sensitivity to context: I. An evolutionary–developmental theory of the origins and functions of stress reactivity.

Development and Psychopathology, 17(2), 271–301. https://doi.org/10.1017/s0954579405050145

Brunton, R. (2022). Child abuse and perinatal outcomes for mother and child: A systematic review of the literature. *Frontiers in Pediatrics*, under review.

Brunton, R., Wood, T., & Dryer, R. (2020). Childhood abuse, pregnancy-related anxiety and the mediating role of resilience and social support. *Journal of Health Psychology, 27*, 868. https://doi.org/10.1177/1359105320968140

Cammack, A. L. (2017). *Child abuse and neglect, preterm birth, and associated mediators.* (Ph.D.). Emory University, Ann Arbor. ProQuest Dissertations & Theses Global database. (10612265).

Cantón-Cortés, D., Cortés, M. R., & Cantón, J. (2012). The role of trauma-genic dynamics on the psychological adjustment of survivors of child sexual abuse. *European Journal of Developmental Psychology, 9*(6), 665–680. https://doi.org/10.1080/17405629.2012.660789

CDC. (2021). *Alcohol use in Pregnancy.* https://www.cdc.gov/ncbddd/fasd/alcohol-use.htm

Chamberlain, C., Ralph, N., Hokke, S., Clark, Y., Gee, G., Stansfield, C., Sutcliffe, K., Brown, S. J., Brennan, S., & Group, H. T. P. B. N. T. F. (2019). Healing the past by nurturing the future: A qualitative systematic review and meta-synthesis of pregnancy, birth and early postpartum experiences and views of parents with a history of childhood maltreatment. *PLoS One, 14*(12), e0225441. https://doi.org/10.1371/journal.pone.0225441

Chawla, N., & Ostafin, B. (2007). Experiential avoidance as a functional dimensional approach to psychopathology: An empirical review. *Journal of Clinical Psychology, 63*(9), 871–890. https://doi.org/10.1002/jclp.20400

Choi, K. W. (2018). *Postpartum depression in the intergenerational transmission of child maltreatment: Longitudinal evidence from global settings.* Dissertation Abstracts International: Section B: The Sciences and Engineering, 78(12-B).

Chung, E. K., Mathew, L., Elo, I. T., Coyne, J. C., & Culhane, J. F. (2008). Depressive symptoms in disadvantaged women receiving prenatal care: The influence of adverse and positive childhood experiences. *Ambulatory Pediatrics, 8*(2), 109–116. https://doi.org/10.1016/j.ambp.2007.12.003

Coe, J. L., Huffhines, L., Gonzalez, D., Seifer, R., & Parade, S. H. (2021). Cascades of risk linking intimate partner violence and adverse childhood experiences to less sensitive caregiving during infancy. *Child Maltreatment, 26*(4), 409–419. https://doi.org/10.1177/10775595211000431

Dietz, P. M., Spitz, A. M., Anda, R. F., Williamson, D. F., McMahon, P. M., Santelli, J. S., Nordenberg, D. F., Felitti, V. J., & Kendrick, J. S. (1999).

Unintended pregnancy among adult women exposed to abuse or household dysfunction during their childhood. *JAMA: Journal of the American Medical Association, 282*(14), 1359. https://doi.org/10.1001/jama.282.14.1359

Drevin, J. (2019). *Measuring pregnancy planning and the effect of childhood abuse on reproductive health.* (Ph.D.). Uppsala Universitet (Sweden), Ann Arbor. http://urn.kb.se/resolve?urn=urn:nbn:se:uu:diva-379739. ProQuest Dissertations & Theses Global database. (13906927).

Eide, J., Hovengen, R., & Nordhagen, R. (2010). Childhood abuse and later worries about the baby's health in pregnancy. *Acta Obstetricia et Gynecologica Scandinavica, 89*(12), 1523–1531. https://doi.org/10.3109/0001634 9.2010.526180

Ellis, B., Boyce, W. T., Belsky, J., Bakermans-Kranenburg, M., & van Ijzendoorn, M. (2011). Differential susceptibility to the environment: An evolutionary–neurodevelopmental theory. *Development and Psychopathology, 23*(1), 7–28. https://doi.org/10.1017/S0954579410000611

Finkelhor, D., & Browne, A. (1985). The traumatic impact of child sexual abuse: A conceptualization. *American Journal of Orthopsychiatry, 55*(4), 530–541.

Garwood, S. K., Gerassi, L., Jonson-Reid, M., Plax, K., & Drake, B. (2015). More than poverty: The effect of child abuse and neglect on teen pregnancy risk. *Journal of Adolescent Health, 57*(2), 164–168. https://doi.org/10.1016/j. jadohealth.2015.05.004

Giovanelli, A., Mondi, C. F., Reynolds, A. J., & Ou, S. R. (2020). Adverse childhood experiences: Mechanisms of risk and resilience in a longitudinal urban cohort. *Development and Psychopathology, 32*(4), 1418–1439. https:// doi.org/10.1017/S095457941900138X

Hayes, S. C., Wilson, K. G., Gifford, E. V., Follette, V. M., & Strosahl, K. (1996). Experiential avoidance and behavioral disorders: A functional dimensional approach to diagnosis and treatment. *Journal of Consulting and Clinical Psychology, 64*(6), 1152. https://doi.org/10.1037/0022-006X.64.6.1152

Hutchens, B. F., Kearney, J., & Kennedy, H. P. (2017). Survivors of child maltreatment and postpartum depression: An integrative review. *Journal of Midwifery & Women's Health, 62*(6), 706–722. https://doi.org/10.1111/ jmwh.12680

Jantzen, K., Ball, S. A., Jantzen, K., Ball, S. A., Leventhal, J. M., & Schottenfeld, R. S. (1998). Types of abuse and cocaine use in pregnant women. *Journal of Substance Abuse Treatment, 15*(4), 319–323. https://doi.org/10.1016/ S0740-5472(97)00198-0

Kallstrom-Fuqua, A. C., Weston, R., & Marshall, L. L. (2004). Childhood and adolescent sexual abuse of community women: Mediated effects on psychological distress and social relationships. *Journal of Consulting & Clinical Psychology, 72*(6), 980. https://doi.org/10.1037/0022-006X.72.6.980

Keegan, J., Parva, M., Finnegan, M., Gerson, A., & Belden, M. (2010). Addiction in pregnancy. *Journal of Addictive Diseases, 29*(2), 175–191. https://doi.org/10.1080/10550881003684723

Kunseler, F. C., Oosterman, M., de Moor, M. H., Verhage, M. L., & Schuengel, C. (2016). Weakened resilience in parenting self-efficacy in pregnant women who were abused in childhood: An experimental test. *PLoS One, 11*(2), e0141801. https://doi.org/10.1371/journal.pone.0141801

Leeners, B., Gorres, G., Block, E., & Hengartner, M. P. (2016). Birth experiences in adult women with a history of childhood sexual abuse. *Journal of Psychosomatic Research, 83,* 27–32. https://doi.org/10.1016/j.jpsychores.2016.02.006

Leeners, B., Neumaier-Wagner, P., Quarg, A. F., & Rath, W. (2006). Childhood sexual abuse (CSA) experiences: An underestimated factor in perinatal care. *Acta Obstetricia et Gynecologica Scandinavica, 85*(8), 971–976. https://doi.org/10.1080/00016340600626917

Leeners, B., Stiller, R., Block, E., Görres, G., Imthurn, B., & Rath, W. (2007). Effect of childhood sexual abuse on gynecologic care as an adult. *Psychosomatics, 48*(5), 385–393. https://doi.org/10.1176/appi.psy.48.5.385

Leeners, B., Stiller, R., Block, E., Gorres, G., Rath, W., & Tschudin, S. (2013). Prenatal care in adult women exposed to childhood sexual abuse. *Journal of Perinatal Medicine, 41*(4), 365–374. https://doi.org/10.1515/jpm-2011-0086

Lev-Wiesel, R., & Daphna-Tekoah, S. (2010). The role of peripartum dissociation as a predictor of posttraumatic stress symptoms following childbirth in Israeli Jewish women. *Journal of Trauma & Dissociation, 11*(3), 266–283. https://doi.org/10.1080/15299731003780887

Littleton, H. (2015). Sexual victimization and somatic complaints in pregnancy: Examination of depression as a mediator. *Women's Health Issues, 25*(6), 696–702. https://doi.org/10.1016/j.whi.2015.06.013

Lukasse, M., Schei, B., Vangen, S., & Oian, P. (2009). Childhood abuse and common complaints in pregnancy. *Birth: Issues in Perinatal Care, 36*(3), 190–199. https://doi.org/10.1111/j.1523-536X.2009.00323.x

Lukasse, M., Vangen, S., Oian, P., Kumle, M., Ryding, E. L., & Schei, B. (2010). Childhood abuse and fear of childbirth—A population-based study. *Birth:*

Issues in Perinatal Care, 37(4), 267–274. https://doi.org/10.1111/j.1523-536X.2010.00420.x

Mahenge, B., Stockl, H., Mizinduko, M., Mazalale, J., & Jahn, A. (2018). Adverse childhood experiences and intimate partner violence during pregnancy and their association to postpartum depression. *Journal of Affective Disorders, 229*, 159–163. https://doi.org/10.1016/j.jad.2017.12.036

Masten, A. S. (2007). Resilience in developing systems: Progress and promise as the fourth wave rises. *Development and Psychopathology, 19*(3), 921–930. https://doi.org/10.1017/s0954579407000442

Masten, A. S., & Cicchetti, D. (2010). Developmental cascades. *Development and Psychopathology, 22*(3), 491–495. https://doi.org/10.1017/S0954579 410000222

Masten, A. S., & Coatsworth, J. D. (1998). The development of competence in favorable and unfavorable environments: Lessons from research on successful children. *American Psychologist, 53*(2), 205. https://doi.org/10.1037/0003-066X.53.2.205

Noll, J. G., Trickett, P. K., & Putnam, F. W. (2003). A prospective investigation of the impact of childhood sexual abuse on the development of sexuality. *Journal of Consulting & Clinical Psychology, 71*(3), 575. https://www.ncbi.nlm.nih.gov/pmc/articles/PMC3012425/pdf/nihms258712.pdf

Plaza, A., Garcia-Esteve, L., Torres, A., Ascaso, C., Gelabert, E., Luisa Imaz, M., Navarro, P., Valdés, M., & Martín-Santos, R. (2012). Childhood physical abuse as a common risk factor for depression and thyroid dysfunction in the earlier postpartum. *Psychiatry Research, 200*(2–3), 329–335. https://doi.org/10.1016/j.psychres.2012.06.032

Post, R. M. (1992). Transduction of psychosocial stress into the neurobiology of recurrent affective disorder. *The American Journal of Psychiatry, 149*, 1727.

Post, R. M. (2016). Epigenetic basis of sensitization to stress, affective episodes, and stimulants: Implications for illness progression and prevention. *Bipolar Disorders, 18*(4), 315–324. https://doi.org/10.1111/bdi.12401

Racine, N., McDonald, S., Chaput, K., Tough, S., & Madigan, S. (2020). Maternal substance use in pregnancy: Differential prediction by childhood adversity subtypes. *Preventive Medicine, 141*, 106303. https://doi.org/10.1016/j.ypmed.2020.106303

Records, K., & Rice, M. J. (2009). Lifetime physical and sexual abuse and the risk for depression symptoms in the first 8 months after birth. *Journal of Psychosomatic Obstetrics and Gynecology, 30*(3), 181–190. https://doi.org/10.1080/01674820903178121

Russotti, J., Handley, E. D., Rogosch, F. A., Toth, S. L., & Cicchetti, D. (2020). The interactive effects of child maltreatment and adolescent pregnancy on late-adolescent depressive symptoms. *Journal of Abnormal Child Psychology, 48*(9), 1223–1237. https://doi.org/10.1007/s10802-020-00669-w

Stroud, C. B., Harkness, K., & Hayden, E. (2020). *The stress sensitization model.* Oxford University Press.

van Breda, A. D. (2018). A critical review of resilience theory and its relevance for social work. *Social Work, 54*, 1–18. https://doi.org/10.15270/54-1-611

Van Ijzendoorn, M. H., & Bakermans-Kranenburg, M. J. (2006). DRD4 7-repeat polymorphism moderates the association between maternal unresolved loss or trauma and infant disorganization. *Attachment & Human Development, 8*(4), 291–307. https://doi.org/10.1080/14616730601048159

Yampolsky, L., Lev-Wiesel, R., & Ben-Zion, I. Z. (2010). Child sexual abuse: Is it a risk factor for pregnancy? *Journal of Advanced Nursing, 66*(9), 2025–2037. https://doi.org/10.1111/j.1365-2648.2010.05387.x

Zhang, X., Sun, J., Wang, J., Chen, Q., Cao, D., Wang, J., & Cao, F. (2020). Suicide ideation among pregnant women: The role of different experiences of childhood abuse. *Journal of Affective Disorders, 266*, 182–186. https://doi.org/10.1016/j.jad.2020.01.119

4

Maltreatment Trauma, Post-traumatic Stress, and the Embodied Experience of Pregnancy and Childbirth of Child Abuse Survivors

Julia Seng (iD)

Abstract When considering the impacts of trauma across the life span, the impacts on the critical window of the childbearing year cannot be overlooked. The trauma of childhood maltreatment is particularly salient to the first pregnancy, as traumatic birth may be to subsequent pregnancies. There are intergenerational patterns of continuity between parents who have histories of childhood maltreatment and abuse and neglect of their children. One in five individuals has experienced childhood maltreatment; although some are resilient, others develop post-traumatic stress disorder (PTSD). The rate of PTSD for those who are pregnant varies, depending on their circumstances. The PTSD rate can be similar to the 4% population rate in affluent perinatal care settings but 14%–32% in racially marginalized clients in disadvantaged settings. In addition to maternal mental health and parenting manifestations, there are physical manifestations associated with PTSD and complex PTSD that are now

J. Seng (✉)
University of Michigan, Ann Arbor, MI, USA
e-mail: julia.seng@survivormoms.org

© The Author(s), under exclusive license to Springer Nature Switzerland AG 2023
R. Brunton, R. Dryer (eds.), *Perinatal Care and Considerations for Survivors of Child Abuse*, https://doi.org/10.1007/978-3-031-33639-3_4

being researched in relation to pregnancy, including allostatic load effects on metabolic, immune, and cardiovascular status. Hypothalamic-pituitary-adrenal (HPA) axis, catecholamines, and oxytocin systems are all implicated in biobehavioral responses. Trauma-related dysregulations in these systems may be mechanisms of lower birthweight, shorter gestation, and loss of breastfeeding. Perinatal clinicians also may observe the fight-or-flight, freeze-or-faint post-traumatic stress reactions associated with reminders of past trauma or "triggers." Addressing "unresolved maternal trauma" ahead of parenting and avoiding retraumatization in the perinatal care relationship are two priority areas for improving perinatal care and outcomes. Perinatal professionals have been focused on depression and anxiety as common perinatal conditions but may only have been seeing the metaphorical tip of the iceberg. The submerged, broad base, in some instances, may be childhood trauma and its post-traumatic sequelae. Building knowledge, skill, and system capacity for integrating trauma-informed care into perinatal services is an opportunity for interprofessional education and teamwork.

Keywords Post-traumatic stress disorder • Perinatal care • Trauma-informed care • Childhood maltreatment • Pregnancy • Midwifery

Seeing Childbearing Through a Post-traumatic Stress Disorder Lens

When considering the impacts of trauma across the life span, the impacts on the critical window of the childbearing year for those who start a family cannot be overlooked. Childhood maltreatment history can affect the childbearing year in particular ways (Sperlich & Seng, 2008). Many survivors are resilient or recovered by the time they start their own families, but a significant proportion live under the shadow of post-traumatic stress sequelae (Alisic et al., 2014). Seeing clients'[1] concerns, needs, and efforts to cope through the lens of post-traumatic stress disorder (PTSD) can help the perinatal care team respond effectively.

---

[1] In this chapter we refer to clients who are expectant and postpartum mothers.

Although healthcare providers will likely want to use the PTSD diagnostic framing, there also are influential non-diagnostic frameworks. Chief among these is the U.S. Substance Abuse and Mental Health Services Administration's (SAMHSA) trauma-informed care (TIC) framework (Huang et al., 2014). The TIC framework defines trauma as three E's (event, experience of it, and effects) rather than as a disorder. It proposes the four R's as vital practice-level behaviors (realizing the ubiquity of trauma among human service clients, recognizing signs and symptoms, responding to these, and focusing particularly on resisting retraumatization). Organizations providing TIC also operate under six key principles: safety; trustworthiness and transparency; peer support; collaboration and mutuality; empowerment and choice; and cultural, historical, and gender issues. The SAMHSA framework and technical assistance are particularly useful in settings that address trauma and PTSD but are not medical in nature (e.g., detention facilities, schools, shelters, and housing services) or that focus on behavioral health. In healthcare settings, including perinatal services, diagnostic language and diagnoses themselves may be primary tools for interprofessional communication and obtaining resources to address client trauma-related needs. The SAMHSA framework can remain useful as a conceptual framing for interpersonal practice, speaking with clients in accessible language, and enhancing the workplace to consider traumatic experiences in work life (trauma-informed care is covered in more detail in Chap. 7.)

PTSD Is a Common Mental Health Condition, Including During Childbearing

Perinatal professionals have been focused on depression and anxiety as common perinatal conditions but may only have been seeing the metaphorical tip of the iceberg. The submerged, broad base may be childhood trauma and its post-traumatic sequelae. Enhancing our focus on PTSD during childbearing has strong potential to improve expectant mothers' experiences and outcomes. Expanding our clinical attention to trauma and PTSD may also improve our own professional satisfaction as we, as clinicians, become more effective by addressing a previously unrecognized problem.

Importantly, the focus on depression and anxiety has not been wrong; rather, it is simply incomplete. Current diagnostic criteria of PTSD include aspects that look like depression and anxiety, that is, low mood or negative cognitions and autonomic hyperarousal, as well as avoidance of reminders, and the hallmark intrusive re-experiencing of the trauma (American Psychiatric Association, 2013; WHO, 2018). PTSD is also comorbid, with full major depressive disorder in approximately half of cases when PTSD becomes chronic (Kessler et al., 1995). Thus, depressed mood, worrying thoughts, and being physically on edge may be the manifestations perceived. But trauma may be a shared root cause. Because it has been taboo to talk about childhood and sexual trauma in particular (Herman, 1992), we have not had a lens to see clearly client struggles with intrusive re-experiencing and avoidance. Nor has it been the habit of perinatal providers to ask about links between current mental health morbidity and past trauma. To complicate matters, prolonged, repeated trauma, like maltreatment, may be shrouded in alterations in awareness and memory and kept secret or walled behind a deep zone of mistrust of others, especially caregivers (Herman, 1992). For these reasons, and because of the significant prevalence and health impact of PTSD, it is incumbent upon clinicians to realize the importance, recognize the signs and symptoms, and respond—including by avoiding retraumatizing clients (Huang et al., 2014).

Across societies, most people have experienced trauma of some type. One in five individuals has experienced childhood maltreatment. The conditional risk of PTSD after interpersonal trauma in childhood is approximately 25% overall, but 33% for girls (Alisic et al., 2014). Women experience PTSD at twice the rate of men. The all-cause (not just maltreatment-related) point-prevalence of PTSD in the general population of women is estimated to be 4.6%–9.7% (Mitchell et al., 2012; Resnick et al., 1993). However, the rate of PTSD for those who are pregnant varies, depending on circumstances. For example, it can be similar to the population rate in affluent samples, but 14%–32% in racially marginalized clients in disadvantaged settings (Gluck et al., 2021; Seng et al., 2009). Women with partial or subclinical PTSD have similar levels of distress and impairment (Stein et al., 2000). During childbearing, even resilient survivors may have lower social support and concerns about keeping their child safe in the context of intergenerational intrafamilial abuse and neglect, consistent with the "loss of resources" model of complex PTSD (Hobfoll et al., 2011; Sperlich & Seng, 2008).

Etiology of PTSD

PTSD is a syndrome with multifactorial causation. Approximately one-third of the risk comes from each of three factors: genetics, family or origin context, and the impact of the trauma exposure itself (Koenen, 2007). The more life-threatening and physically intrusive the trauma, the greater the risk. In families with multiple generations of maltreatment, and in members of cultural groups with decades or centuries of historical trauma, the risk is even higher (Harnett & Ressler, 2021). But we are learning from the field of epigenetics that biology is not destiny. Maternal caregiving can effectively bend the arc of both individual outcomes and population health, changing both offspring mental health and development and the traits the offspring generation passes on to their offspring (Weaver et al., 2004).

Childhood Maltreatment and PTSD: An Embodied View of PTSD and Complex PTSD

Post-traumatic stress, especially the complex PTSD that is rooted in childhood maltreatment, affects the mind and body, as well as relationships (Herman, 1992; van der Kolk, 2014). If we take in a narrative understanding that the child suffering chronic abuse or neglect or both adapts to survive, it is easier to observe the adaptations. Mental health professionals tend to prioritize focus on the mental manifestations of trauma sequelae. Healthcare professionals could likely be equally effective addressing the physical manifestations. In primary care, the physical morbidity associated with PTSD and complex PTSD includes chronic pain, somatic dysregulations such as irritable bowel syndrome, and ultimately a shortened life span due to metabolic, immune, and cardiovascular conditions (Felitti et al., 1998; Herzog & Schmahl, 2018; Seng et al., 2013a). Lower birth weight and shorter gestation are known outcomes of PTSD in pregnancy (Sanjuan et al., 2021; Seng et al., 2011). Other physical manifestations of maltreatment-related PTSD (e.g., hyperemesis, loss of breastfeeding) have been theorized and reported in small studies (Eagen-Torkko et al., 2017; Seng et al., 2013a); however, systematic research to fully characterize the embodied experience of pregnancy with PTSD, from symptoms to the allostatic load that causes metabolic, immune, and cardiovascular morbidity, remains to be undertaken.

A major conceptualization of PTSD is that it reflects the failure of extinction of the fear response (in "deficit" language) or maintenance of readiness to self-protect at any moment (Pitman et al., 2001). Fight-or-flight sympathetic nervous system responses reset homeostatic mechanisms to a higher level of readiness that can become an allostatic overload (McEwen & Stellar, 1993). Essentially the hypothalamic-pituitary-adrenal (HPA) axis works at a higher baseline and keeps the metabolic, cardiovascular, respiratory, and immune systems "revving" to be ready for danger all the time. This is coupled with behavioral and cognitive avoidance of any reminders of the trauma that can trigger fight-or-flight. In terms of client behavior, we see startle reactions, anger or combative stances, impulsiveness, and efforts to control situations. These fight-or-flight systems and avoidance efforts are predominant in "classic" PTSD, that is, PTSD occurring from single-episode or adulthood trauma exposures.

Freeze or faint reactions occur too. These naturally occur *during* any traumatic event and in the weeks of aftermath and recovery. But in 14% of people with PTSD, these peritraumatic reactions become overgeneralized and part of a complex PTSD or dissociative subtype of PTSD (Stein et al., 2013). Dissociative depersonalization or derealization (i.e., feeling out-of-body or like what is happening is not real) was for an abused child the escape when there is no escape (Putnam, 1992). But dissociation can be carried into adulthood and occur in response to stress, feeling overwhelmed, or reminders of trauma (i.e., triggers). Dissociation in labor occurs among a minority of maltreatment survivors. It can be useful to think of dissociation in labor as a "state," with "trait" or pre-existing dissociation a predisposing factor (Choi & Seng, 2016). Although less is known of the physiology of freeze or faint responses, dissociation is thought to be a parasympathetic response, a form of self-anesthesia when injury or death is unavoidable. These reactions may be based in the oxytocin system (Porges, 2011).

Perinatal professionals are most familiar with oxytocin, which functions on smooth muscles engaged in orgasm, uterine contractions, and milk ejection. Oxytocin is also a neurotransmitter engaged in stress reduction, pro-social, caregiving, and pair bond relationships, and the daily functions that help species, including humans, to thrive: play, exploration, relationships, digesting, growing, and wound healing (Moberg & Moberg, 2003).

Cascade theory tells us that a maltreated child experiences a series of physiological adaptations in cascading order, from oxytocin system to HPA axis and catecholamines (Teicher et al., 2003). In a healthy state, these systems are mutually regulating. In clients with maltreatment-related PTSD, it is useful to think that these body systems are likely mutually *dys*regulated. Much more perinatal research is needed, but theory is useful as a lens. If anger or fear (fight-or-flight) is sensed in client behavior or felt in the client-provider relationship, might we also see HPA-mediated physical alterations? If there is mistrust, a lack of ability to rest, be calm, or care for the self, a sense of disconnection or "surrender" in labor (Rhodes & Hutchinson, 1994), might we also see oxytocin-mediated physical alterations? We have long known that stress responses disrupt labor progress. Using a trauma and PTSD lens, this view can extend to watch for relational challenges in perinatal care and make sense of problems in pregnancy, labor, breastfeeding, and parenting that may be oxytocin mediated.

PTSD and dissociation are also associated with amnesia for all or part of the trauma. This amnesia can begin to subside in adulthood as the utility of knowing what happened to them as a child becomes greater than the utility of not knowing (Freyd, 1996). Major life events, such as the death of a perpetrator or becoming a parent, are known to cause this balance to shift. Triggers are also known to cause this balance to shift (Freyd, 1996; Herman, 1992). Thus, birth attendants may be present at significant moments of loss of amnesia—flashbacks, sudden realizations that they remember a trauma—and so birth attendants may witness the delayed onset of PTSD. Perinatal providers who recognize this trauma reaction are in a position to turn a horrible moment into a healing one (Sperlich & Seng, 2008).

In addition to thinking about PTSD and complex PTSD in terms of mutually regulating and dysregulating hormones, functional neuroimaging studies shed light on brain patterns that are useful as well. In PTSD reactions, where fight-or-flight dominates, we see *under-modulation* (i.e., assessment of the reality of the situation goes offline, and we prepare to ensure survival if we can) of fear reactions. In complex PTSD reactions characterized by dissociation and freeze or faint responses, we see *over-modulation* (i.e., the brain is working to mute the response, playing dead to survive or self-anesthetizing to be numb to the death blow) of fear reactions (Lanius et al., 2010).

These embodied post-traumatic reactions are noxious. People with PTSD are known to try to mute the symptoms with substances or self-harming behaviors as efforts at self-medication (Hawn et al., 2020). In pregnancy clinicians see clients they are concerned about—those smoking, drinking, using drugs, overeating, and with violent partners—are strongly clustered among those with PTSD (Morland et al., 2007; Seng et al., 2008). Trauma-informed perinatal care (described below) may be more successful than earlier approaches for mitigating addiction and family violence that have not considered trauma or post-traumatic stress as the root cause of the presenting problem (Morland et al., 2007).

Other Sources of Perinatal PTSD

PTSD that is activated in pregnancy can have roots in trauma exposures other than maltreatment. Previous medical trauma, prior perinatal loss, or traumatic birth all have the potential to trigger PTSD during subsequent pregnancies. It is important to realize that there is a potential overlap between childhood trauma and subsequent trauma exposure and risk for PTSD from the subsequent exposure. So, some perinatal or medical trauma survivors may also be survivors of childhood trauma with more complex presentations. This can be illustrated from research on PTSD following childbirth, that is, PTSD occurring postpartum, where the birth experience was the ostensible trauma exposure. Childhood sexual abuse and prior psychiatric treatment are known predisposing factors for experiencing birth as traumatic and becoming symptomatic with PTSD (Ayers et al., 2016; Grekin & O'Hara, 2014). Subjective experience, including perceiving the care in labor as uncaring or incompetent (i.e., negligent or abusive), is also a precipitating factor, as well as obstetric emergencies and instrumented or surgical deliveries (Czarnocka & Slade, 2000; Dikmen-Yildiz et al., 2017). But in prospective research, among those who exhibit full PTSD postpartum, most individuals appear to have had PTSD prenatally, and a minority have new-onset PTSD (Seng et al., 2013b).

PTSD and Disparities

There is a saying, "If it's not racially just, it's not trauma-informed" (Dhaliwal, 2016, Fig. 1). PTSD in pregnancy and adverse birth outcomes both occur at much higher rates in cultural groups that experience racism, discrimination, or other forms of marginalization. Rates of childhood maltreatment are similar across racial groups, but rates of resilience are lower, as are resources for recovery (Seng et al., 2011). Although the focus of this chapter is on intergenerational trauma in the form of childhood maltreatment, it is likely that cumulative, multigenerational trauma in the form of racism also contributes to risk for PTSD (Conching & Thayer, 2019), as well as risk for adverse perinatal outcomes (Sotero, 2006). The toll is not only in the form of stressed relationships between minority clients and most often dominant-culture healthcare providers and less satisfying prenatal and birth care, it is also manifested in the bodily health status of minority clients. Traumatic stress, that is pervasive and ongoing, causes premature aging (i.e., weathering) (Geronimus,

1992; Jones et al., 2019). It may also make minority women more vulnerable to having the demands of pregnancy on the body tip allostatic overload into manifesting disease and affecting the fetus. Active changes to practice and systems are needed (Hardeman et al., 2020; Scott et al., 2019), as is research to learn what trauma-informed, equitable, and antiracist care can do to mitigate the syndemic effects of trauma, racism, and PTSD.

PTSD and Perinatal Providers' Trauma

Of course, providers and other perinatal team members are subject to trauma and PTSD as well. This can be either from childhood maltreatment or secondary to work-related traumatic events (e.g., Slade et al., 2020) or both. Failure of fear extinction or maintaining readiness to self-protect at any moment (whether a danger is present or not) may be a post-traumatic manifestation affecting perinatal providers too. Work-related trauma exposure and vicarious trauma are almost inevitable exposures in this field. Yet there is scant support for clinicians to honor our needs to recover and return to a healthy level of vigilance rather than to respond with persistent fight-or-flight and avoidance that may affect our practice. The U.S. Substance Abuse and Mental Health services Administration (SAMHSA) framework for trauma-informed care emphasizes the clients' needs. It only addresses secondarily the providers may have trauma-related needs too and that these should be considered in systems change efforts (Huang et al., 2014). Another influential definition of trauma-informed care proposed by Hopper et al. (2010) makes the need for balancing attention to clients and providers more explicit:

> Trauma-informed care is a strengths based framework that is grounded in an understanding of and responsiveness to the impact of trauma, that emphasizes physical, psychological and emotional safety *for both providers and survivors* [emphasis added], and that creates opportunities for survivors to rebuild a sense of control and empowerment. (p. 82)

PTSD and Complex PTSD Diagnostic Criteria

In a trauma-informed system of perinatal care, it will sometimes be necessary to refer clients (or clinicians) to mental health professionals who can provide evidence-based treatments for PTSD (Forbes et al., 2020; Ford & Courtois, 2020). Diagnosis of PTSD and complex PTSD is not necessary to respond to client needs at the bedside in perinatal care. However, knowing the vocabulary and criteria for diagnosing may help make referrals. In places where mental healthcare specific to PTSD is scarce, consultation or teamwork may be enhanced by speaking the same language.

DSM-5 and ICD-11 have more similarities than differences, as shown in Table 4.1 (American Psychiatric Association, 2013; WHO, 2018). DSM-5 defines a trauma criterion, four PTSD symptom clusters, and it is possible to add a dissociative subtype specifier. The fourth symptoms cluster, not shared with ICD-11, involves exaggerated negative beliefs or persistent negative emotions. ICD-11 PTSD diagnosis requires symptoms in three clusters shared with the DSM-5 (i.e., intrusions and re-experiencing, avoidance, and arousal and reactivity). For complex PTSD, ICD-11 requires these three, and three more, symptoms considered to reflect disorganization of the self (i.e., affect dysregulation, negative beliefs about oneself, difficulty sustaining relationships). These are not entirely different from the fourth DSM-5 PTSD cluster. Both taxonomies require significant distress and impairment in role functioning as well.

The Role of Perinatal Care Team Members in Addressing PTSD During the Childbearing Year

While it is not generally the role of perinatal care providers to treat PTSD, we are beginning to know that they *do* need to step up to address unmet maltreatment—or PTSD-related needs (Nagle-Yang et al., 2022). The question at this time is how to conceptualize this work, create approaches or interventions, and study their effects.

Table 4.1 Comparison of DSM-5 and ICD-11 criteria for diagnosis of PTSD and complex PTSD

Source	Criterion
Both DSM-5 and ICD-11	*Trauma exposure* DSM-5: Exposure to actual or threatened death, serious injury, or sexual violence ICD-11: Exposure to extremely threatening or horrific event or series of events
Both DSM-5 and ICD-11	*Intrusions or re-experiencing of the event* (such as intrusive memories, repetitive play in which the events or aspects of it are expressed, nightmares, flashbacks, distress triggered by reminders of the event or events) *Avoidance* (such as avoiding thoughts, feelings or memories of the event or events, or avoiding people, places, conversations, or situations that are associated with the event or the events) *Arousal and reactivity* or sense of current threat (such as irritability, being overly vigilant, being easily startled, concentration problems, sleep problems)
Additional DSM-5 criterion for PTSD	*Exaggerated negative beliefs* about themselves, the world, or other people; having distorted thoughts about what caused the event or events and the consequences; *or persistent negative emotions*; less interest in significant events; feeling detached or estranged from others and finding it impossible to experience positive emotions
Additional ICD-11 criteria for Complex PTSD (CPTSD)	*Problems in affect regulation* (such as marked irritability or anger, feeling emotionally numb) *Beliefs about oneself* as diminished, defeated, or worthless, accompanied by feelings of shame, guilt or failure related to the traumatic event *Difficulties in sustaining relationships* and in feeling close to others
DSM-5 specifier for dissociative subtype (PTSD-D)	*Definition of dissociation generally*: a disruption, interruption, and/or discontinuity of the normal, subjective integration of behavior, memory, identity, consciousness, emotion, perception, body representation, and motor control. *Depersonalization and derealization* specifically: Experiences of unreality, detachment, or being an outside observer with respect to one's thoughts, feelings, sensations, body, or actions (e.g., perceptual alterations, distorted sense of time, unreal or absent self, emotional and/or physical numbing).

Table 4.1 is modified from the comparative explanation on the UK Trauma Council website, https://uktraumacouncil.org/trauma/ptsd-and-complex-ptsd accessed 6 August 2022 and from the WHO ICD-11 and American Psychiatric Association DSM-5

There are perhaps many ways to conceptualize, but theory and qualitative research suggest two imperatives clinicians can address. The first involves three of the four R's of the trauma-informed approach: "realize, recognize, and respond." In perinatal care, this can take the shape of becoming an ally to the person as they name, understand, and start to work on any "unresolved maternal trauma" that may be affecting them. The second involves the fourth R: resisting retraumatizing. (Note that Chap. 6 explains trauma-informed care in more depth.)

A First Imperative: To Address "Unresolved Maternal Trauma" Ahead of Parenting

Women psychoanalysts from the middle of the twentieth century, Helene Deutsch and Greta Bibring, noted that childhood maltreatment trauma loomed large when their survivor patients became pregnant and that therapy during pregnancy progressed very well (Bibring, 1959; Deutsch, 1945). By the 1970s, this phenomenon was referred to by Selma Fraiberg and others as "ghosts in the nursery" and "unresolved maternal trauma" (Fraiberg et al., 1975). These threads of thought have been carried forward by contemporary psychology writers, but in works more often of use to psychotherapists than to perinatal healthcare providers (e.g., Raphael-Leff, 2018; Weinstein, 2016).

Qualitative reports have included statements from women's perspectives that tell the same story, but in simpler words. They often realized at some level during pregnancy that their maltreatment history presented challenges to becoming a parent that they felt compelled to confront "right now" (Sperlich & Seng, 2008). In a nutshell, they wanted to stop the cycle of maltreatment and become a good-enough parent (i.e., sensitive, reflective, safe) in time to raise a child in a better way than they were raised. When asked what they wanted maternity care providers to do, their answers varied based on where they were in the recovery process. Generally, they wanted to know they were not the only one, that maternity care providers would be allies in this effort, would address their risk behaviors in a trauma-informed way, and would lay the groundwork for getting mental health treatment at some point, when they were ready or if their trauma coping became overwhelmed by childbearing. They wanted perinatal caregivers to focus on addressing their trauma for the sake of having a positive birth experience and acquiring solid maternal role development despite the shadow of maltreatment trauma (Seng et al., 2002).

So, a first conceptualization of the role of perinatal providers could be that of allies in the metaphorical act of turning a light on to banish the ghosts in the nursery. This won't be an overnight accomplishment. But naming the issues; providing information, skills, and emotional support; and being in a relationship are practices that can be deployed from within our scope of practice.

The caregiver role with an infant involves dyadic emotion regulation and providing a secure holding environment (Rowe et al., 2015). Any perinatal client, especially those having a first birth, may need this sort of generativity from the midwife or obstetrician during moments of vulnerability or uncertainty. Clinicians probably do this without any special attention to such exchanges. For clients who have survived maltreatment, these normal moments of vulnerability or uncertainty may feel intense and trigger symptoms of PTSD. If they become symptomatic, we can expect them to be physically dysregulated during fight-flight-freeze reactions or by hypervigilance and to have feelings of being in danger and needing to be mistrustful. If we can imagine the lack of dyadic emotion regulation and secure holding that survivors may have received as a young child, it suggests these maternal tasks could be used as templates for useful responses to clients (Rowe et al., 2015). We can help them regulate emotions that are out of proportion to what is happening. We can give them a safe space in which to express fears of what lies ahead and doubts about themselves and provide encouragement. But to do this, we must be aware of clients' trauma history and the extent of their post-traumatic mental health sequelae. And we have to have a practice environment that supports the work within the six key principles of a trauma-informed approach applied to the workforce as well as clients.

A Second Imperative: To Provide Perinatal Care that Resists Retraumatization

The work of supporting clients with maltreatment history is not at all likely to succeed if we (as clinicians) cannot resist retraumatization. At its most basic, retraumatizing a maltreatment survivor involves acting or relating in a manner that *is* similar to, or that is perceived to be similar to, the acts or relational behavior of the perpetrator of the original abuse or neglect.

Neither the healthcare system nor the staff want to think of their environment, routines, or ways of relating as traumagenic. But we need only look through the lenses of childhood maltreatment to see blatant and subtle ways in which the context and behaviors that we accept as normal have the potential to retraumatize those who have experienced sexual abuse, physical abuse, physical neglect, emotional abuse, or emotional neglect at the hands of caregivers. The clinical literature has examples of how internal examinations can retraumatize sexual abuse survivors (e.g., Rose, 1992) and also suggestions for how to change the environment, actions, and relational dynamic to be collaborative and empowering (e.g., Simkin & Klaus, 2004). Examples for the latter include providing progressive, repeated rather than one-time or assumed informed consent and asking for permission to conduct an internal examination of their body, providing chaperones, and asking about preferences for privacy, positioning, and draping. Explaining what a trigger is and asking clients if they have noticed things that trigger them, then collaborating to make plans to avoid those triggers is another example.

In perinatal care, we do not focus as much on retraumatization related to physical abuse. It is not hard to see though that environments and practice behaviors that diminish dignity, humiliate, and show disregard for pain or the need for body integrity could be retraumatizing. An example could be the medical routine of having patients undress and sit on the exam table, waiting for the provider to enter the room, which can resemble the experience of a child waiting in their room for a parent to arrive and use corporal punishment. Neglect of physical needs occurs as well, though we may not give it that name. For example, from the perspective of a maltreatment survivor, having food and water withheld in labor, being required to wear an inadequate gown, or having needed support withheld inequitably (e.g., having epidural anesthesia or lactation help or doula support depends on insured status or location of the hospital) would be likely to anger or disempower them. It is true that any person might be adversely affected by these experiences; maltreatment survivors with post-traumatic sequelae may experience PTSD reactions that are distressing and impair their ability to question authorities or advocate for themselves.

More subtle, perhaps, but no less important, is the potential for emotional abuse and neglect to happen or be perceived in client-provider-team relationships. So, providers who ignore or dismiss survivors' needs may be triggering survivors to engage in fight-or-flight, freeze or faint reactions rather than strengthening them to engage purposefully in mutual collaboration to address the trauma and resist retraumatization together.

Two theories of what causes PTSD or complex PTSD are relational theories. Judith Herman's (1992) point that maltreatment is an injury to the attachment system and Jennifer Freyd's (1996) view that it is a betrayal can guide providers and staff to focus on the quality of their caring. If we know that the provider relationship is significant for the client—one where they will be vulnerable and need our care in a time of pain and existential transition—then we can strive to be trustworthy and reliably connected. If we understand how betrayal traumatizes, we can be transparent about limitations, shortcomings, or injustices and form alliances with clients to advocate, call out, and work for change.

Providers cannot carry the responsibility of resisting retraumatization alone. The needs of pregnant and early parenting survivors can be numerous and complex if we see them fully and assess for them systematically. Needs can include mental health, substance use, violence-related services, parenting education, social support, and care for the physical health decrements that are found with PTSD. It is worth this comprehensive psychosocial and health status assessment if we want to see improvements in the health of individual parents, children of the next generation, and the overall population. But this would require political will to add resources and redesign our service delivery models to be trauma-informed and address perinatal and post-traumatic needs in tandem.

Where to Begin? Structure, Process, Outcome

Achieving changes to outcomes can require changes at the systems level (White & Griffith, 2019), requiring attention to existing structures and processes and planning modifications or adaptations to achieve the preferred outcomes. Interprofessional work in perinatal services—where physical, psychosocial, and mental health services are integrated—provides a structure that should be capable of providing care adequate to address perinatal needs rooted in maltreatment-related trauma holistically. The process of change may be slow. Perinatal pathways to specialist mental health treatment may not currently include evidence-based treatment for PTSD (which still lacks evidence for safety during pregnancy) (Baas et al., 2020; Stevens et al., 2021). Screening efforts may not yet be smooth. A "don't ask, don't tell" mindset will prevail if there are not feasible, acceptable, or satisfying offerings in response to disclosure. It will take a process of trial, error, evaluation, revision, and success to get to a point where the team is confident in what they can do for survivors—at universal, targeted, and specialist levels. The outcomes will be both easy and hard to see. Based on theory, addressing post-traumatic stress and other sequelae from childhood maltreatment should yield a host of population health improvements, none of which may be evident at the individual level. Pregnancy PTSD is associated with shorter gestation and lower birth weight, less breastfeeding despite a greater intention to breastfeed, a greater burden from traumatic birth and postpartum PTSD and depression, impaired bonding, and difficulties in infant regulation and development (Eagen-Torkko et al., 2017; Enlow et al., 2011; Sanjuan et al., 2021; Seng et al., 2013b). Pregnancy PTSD may also be a critical intra-uterine transmission point for life span health risks conceptualized as developmental origins of health and disease (Seng et al., 2018). But it would take quantifiable interventions and large-scale research to model the impact of trauma-informed perinatal care on most of these outcomes.

We could make a start on this. But we cannot wait for evidence of the impact on the population.

At the individual level, evaluation of our interventions—practice behaviors and programs or treatments—might suffice to indicate we are going in the right direction. Proximal outcomes such as positive appraisals of experience, satisfying ratings of alliance and relationships, decreased burden of perinatal mental health and substance use, increased parenting sense of competence, and ability to enjoy the postpartum period are all potential good outcomes for clients. For providers, growth in competence, shared trauma-informed work, shared triumphs in system changes, and even our own personal increase in professional quality of life are potential good outcomes (Geoffrion et al., 2019). All these—client and provider outcomes—have measurable indicators that would be sensitive to change at a reasonable time in the future.

A Hallmark of Trauma-Informed Change for the Perinatal Professions

A change in a staff member's habit of mind is a commonly understood hallmark of trauma-informed mental health and addiction care. This shift is from wondering about a client, "What is *wrong* with you?" to wondering "What *happened* to you?" There may be a similarly brief way to state what could be a hallmark of trauma-informed perinatal care. We would be enacting a trauma-informed approach in perinatal care if we shifted from locating the problem in the client as "*unresolved* maternal trauma" to locating it in our system and professional care as "*unaddressed* maternal trauma."

We can use mind-body and relational understandings of maltreatment-related post-traumatic stress to spot physical, psychological, and maternal development problems rooted in childhood trauma. We have expertise in the bodily experiences of pregnancy, birth, breastfeeding, and early parenting. We can name the numerous sequelae of maltreatment trauma that impinge on good childbearing processes and outcomes as significant clinical problems. We can state the reality that some responses are indeed within our domain as childbearing care providers—and make it so. We can make a claim for adequate resources and a trauma-informed system of perinatal services. We cannot control whether our care will have the effect of fully resolving any individual's unresolved maternal trauma, but we can take some control over whether we have addressed it well.

References

Alisic, E., Zalta, A. K., Van Wesel, F., Larsen, S. E., Hafstad, G. S., Hassanpour, K., & Smid, G. E. (2014). Rates of post-traumatic stress disorder in trauma-exposed children and adolescents: Meta-analysis. *The British Journal of Psychiatry, 204*(5), 335–340. https://doi.org/10.1192/bjp.bp.113.131227

American Psychiatric Association. (2013). *Diagnostic and statistical manual of mental disorders* (5th ed.). American Psychiatric Association.

Ayers, S., Bond, R., Bertullies, S., & Wijma, K. (2016). The aetiology of post-traumatic stress following childbirth: A meta-analysis and theoretical framework. *Psychological Medicine, 46*(6), 1121–1134. https://doi.org/10.1017/S0033291715002706

Baas, M. A., van Pampus, M. G., Braam, L., Stramrood, C. A., & de Jongh, A. (2020). The effects of PTSD treatment during pregnancy: Systematic review and case study. *European Journal of Psychotraumatology, 11*(1), 1762310. https://doi.org/10.1080/20008198.2020.1762310

Bibring, G. L. (1959). Some considerations of the psychological processes in pregnancy. *The Psychoanalytic Study of the Child, 14*, 113–121. https://doi.org/10.1080/00797308.1959.11822824

Choi, K. R., & Seng, J. S. (2016). Predisposing and precipitating factors for dissociation during labor in a cohort study of posttraumatic stress disorder and childbearing outcomes. *Journal of Midwifery & Women's Health, 61*(1), 68–76. https://doi.org/10.1111/jmwh.12364

Conching, A. K. S., & Thayer, Z. (2019). Biological pathways for historical trauma to affect health: A conceptual model focusing on epigenetic modifications. *Social Science & Medicine, 230*, 74–82. https://doi.org/10.1016/j.socscimed.2019.04.001

Czarnocka, J., & Slade, P. (2000). Prevalence and predictors of post-traumatic stress symptoms following childbirth. *British Journal of Clinical Psychology, 39*(1), 35–51. https://doi.org/10.1348/014466500163095

Deutsch, H. (1945). *The psychology of women* (Vol. 2). Grune & Stratton.

Dhaliwal, K. (2016, October 24). Racing ACEs gathering and reflection: If it's not racially just, it's not trauma-informed. *ACES Too High* blog post. https://acestoohigh.com/2016/10/24/racing-aces-gathering-and-reflection-if-its-not-racially-just-its-not-trauma-informed/

Dikmen-Yildiz, P., Ayers, S., & Phillips, L. (2017). Factors associated with post-traumatic stress symptoms (PTSS) 4-6 weeks and 6 months after birth: A longitudinal population-based study. *Journal of Affective Disorders, 221*, 238–245. https://doi.org/10.1016/j.jad.2017.06.049

Eagen-Torkko, M., Low, L. K., Zielinski, R., & Seng, J. S. (2017). Prevalence and predictors of breastfeeding after childhood abuse. *Journal of Obstetric, Gynecologic & Neonatal Nursing, 46*(3), 465–479. https://doi.org/10.1016/j.jogn.2017.01.002

Enlow, M. B., Kitts, R. L., Blood, E., Bizarro, A., Hofmeister, M., & Wright, R. J. (2011). Maternal posttraumatic stress symptoms and infant emotional reactivity and emotion regulation. *Infant Behavior and Development, 34*(4), 487–503. https://doi.org/10.1016/j.infbeh.2011.07.007

Felitti, V. J., Anda, R. F., Nordenberg, D., Williamson, D. F., Spitz, A. M., Edwards, V., & Marks, J. S. (1998). Relationship of childhood abuse and household dysfunction to many of the leading causes of death in adults: The Adverse Childhood Experiences (ACE) Study. *American Journal of Preventive Medicine, 14*(4), 245–258. https://doi.org/10.1016/s0749-3797(98)00017-8

Forbes, D., Bisson, J. I., Monson, C. M., & Berliner, L. (Eds.). (2020). *Effective treatments for PTSD.* Guilford Publications.

Ford, J. D., & Courtois, C. A. (2020). *Treating complex traumatic stress disorders in adults: Scientific foundations and therapeutic models.* Guilford Publications.

Fraiberg, S., Adelson, E., & Shapiro, V. (1975). Ghosts in the nursery: A psychoanalytic approach to the problems of impaired infant–mother relationships. *Journal of the American Academy of Child Psychiatry, 14*(3), 387–421. https://doi.org/10.1016/S0002-7138(09)61442-4

Freyd, J. J. (1996). *Betrayal trauma: The logic of forgetting childhood abuse.* Harvard University Press.

Geoffrion, S., Lamothe, J., Morizot, J., & Giguère, C. É. (2019). Construct validity of the professional quality of life (ProQoL) scale in a sample of child protection workers. *Journal of Traumatic Stress, 32*(4), 566–576. https://doi.org/10.1002/jts.22410

Geronimus, A. T. (1992). The weathering hypothesis and the health of African-American women and infants: Evidence and speculations. *Ethnicity & Disease, 2*(3), 207–221.

Gluck, R. L., Hartzell, G. E., Dixon, H. D., Michopoulos, V., Powers, A., Stevens, J. S., Fani, N., Carter, S., Schwartz, A. C., Jovanovic, T., Ressler, K. J., Bradley, B., & Gillespie, C. F. (2021). Trauma exposure and stress-related disorders in a large, urban, predominantly African-American, female sample. *Archives of Women's Mental Health, 24*(6), 893–901. https://doi. org/10.1007/s00737-021-01141-4

Grekin, R., & O'Hara, M. W. (2014). Prevalence and risk factors of postpartum posttraumatic stress disorder: A meta-analysis. *Clinical Psychology Review, 34*(5), 389–401. https://doi.org/10.1016/j.cpr.2014.05.003

Hardeman, R. R., Karbeah, J. M., & Kozhimannil, K. B. (2020). Applying a critical race lens to relationship-centered care in pregnancy and childbirth: An antidote to structural racism. *Birth, 47*(1), 3–7. https://doi.org/10.1111/ birt.12462

Harnett, N. G., & Ressler, K. J. (2021). Structural racism as a proximal cause for race-related differences in psychiatric disorders. *American Journal of Psychiatry, 178*(7), 579–581. https://doi.org/10.1176/appi.ajp.2021.21050486

Hawn, S. E., Cusack, S. E., & Amstadter, A. B. (2020). A systematic review of the self-medication hypothesis in the context of posttraumatic stress disorder and comorbid problematic alcohol use. *Journal of Traumatic Stress, 33*(5), 699–708. https://doi.org/10.1002/jts.22521

Herman, J. L. (1992). *Trauma and recovery*. Basic Books.

Herzog, J. I., & Schmahl, C. (2018). Adverse childhood experiences and the consequences on neurobiological, psychosocial, and somatic conditions across the lifespan. *Frontiers in Psychiatry, 9*, 420. https://doi.org/10.3389/ fpsyt.2018.00420

Hobfoll, S. E., Mancini, A. D., Hall, B. J., Canetti, D., & Bonanno, G. A. (2011). The limits of resilience: Distress following chronic political violence among Palestinians. *Social Science & Medicine, 72*(8), 1400–1408. https://doi. org/10.1016/j.socscimed.2011.02.022

Hopper, K., Bassuk, E., & Olivet, J. (2010). Shelter from the storm: Trauma-informed care in homelessness services settings. *The Open Health Services and Policy Journal, 3*(1), 80–100. https://doi.org/10.2174/ 1874924001003010080

Huang, L. N., Flatow, R., Biggs, T., Afayee, S., Smith, K., Clark, T., & Blake, M. (2014). *SAMHSA's concept of trauma and guidance for a trauma-informed approach.*

Jones, N. L., Gilman, S. E., Cheng, T. L., Drury, S. S., Hill, C. V., & Geronimus, A. T. (2019). Life course approaches to the causes of health disparities.

American Journal of Public Health, 109(S1), S48–S55. https://doi. org/10.2105/AJPH.2018.304738

Kessler, R. C., Sonnega, A., Bromet, E., Hughes, M., & Nelson, C. B. (1995). Posttraumatic stress disorder in the National Comorbidity Survey. *Archives of General Psychiatry, 52*(12), 1048–1060. https://doi.org/10.1001/ archpsyc.1995.03950240066012

Koenen, K. C. (2007). Genetics of posttraumatic stress disorder: Review and recommendations for future studies. *Journal of Traumatic Stress, 20*(5), 737–750. https://doi.org/10.1002/jts.20205

Lanius, R. A., Vermetten, E., Loewenstein, R. J., Brand, B., Schmahl, C., Bremner, J. D., & Spiegel, D. (2010). Emotion modulation in PTSD: Clinical and neurobiological evidence for a dissociative subtype. *American Journal of Psychiatry, 167*(6), 640–647. https://doi.org/10.1176/appi. ajp.2009.09081168

McEwen, B. S., & Stellar, E. (1993). Stress and the individual: Mechanisms leading to disease. *Archives of Internal Medicine, 153*(18), 2093–2101. https://doi.org/10.1001/archinte.1993.00410180039004

Mitchell, K. S., Mazzeo, S. E., Schlesinger, M. R., Brewerton, T. D., & Smith, B. N. (2012). Comorbidity of partial and subthreshold PTSD among men and women with eating disorders in the National Comorbidity Survey-Replication Study. *International Journal of Eating Disorders, 45*, 307–315. https://doi.org/10.1002/eat.20965

Moberg, K. U., & Moberg, K. (2003). *The oxytocin factor: Tapping the hormone of calm, love, and healing*. Da Capo Press.

Morland, L., Goebert, D., Onoye, J., Frattarelli, L., Derauf, C., Herbst, M., Matsu, C., & Friedman, M. (2007). Posttraumatic stress disorder and pregnancy health: Preliminary update and implications. *Psychosomatics, 48*(4), 304–308. https://doi.org/10.1176/appi.psy.48.4.304

Nagle-Yang, S., Sachdeva, J., Zhao, L. X., Shenai, N., Shirvani, N., Worley, L. L., Gopalan, P., Albertini, E. S., Spada, M., Mittal, L., Moore Simas, T. A., & Byatt, N. (2022). Trauma-informed care for obstetric and gynecologic settings. *Maternal and Child Health Journal, 26*, 2362–2369. https://doi. org/10.1007/s10995-022-03518-y

Pitman, R. K., Shin, L. M., & Rauch, S. L. (2001). Investigating the pathogenesis of posttraumatic stress disorder with neuroimaging. *Journal of Clinical Psychiatry, 62*(Suppl 17), 47–54.

Porges, S. W. (2011). *The polyvagal theory: Neurophysiological foundations of emotions, attachment, communication, and self-regulation (Norton series on interpersonal neurobiology)*. W. W. Norton & Company.

Putnam, F. W. (1992). Discussion: Are alter personalities fragments or figments? *Psychoanalytic Inquiry, 12*, 95.

Raphael-Leff, J. (2018). *The psychological processes of childbearing*. Routledge.

Resnick, H. S., Kilpatrick, D. G., Dansky, B. S., Saunders, B. E., & Best, C. L. (1993). Prevalence of civilian trauma and posttraumatic stress disorder in a representative national sample of women. *Journal of Consulting and Clinical Psychology, 61*(6), 984. https://doi.org/10.1037/0022-006X.61.6.984

Rhodes, N., & Hutchinson, S. (1994). Labor experiences of childhood sexual abuse survivors. *Birth, 21*(4), 213–220. https://doi.org/10.1111/j.1523-536X.1994.tb00532.x

Rose, A. (1992). Effects of childhood sexual abuse on childbirth: One woman's story. *Birth, 19*(4), 214–218.

Rowe, H., Seng, J., Acton, C., & Fisher, J. (2015). The postnatal period-opportunities for creating change. In *Trauma informed care in the perinatal period* (pp. 74–92). Academic Press.

Sanjuan, P. M., Fokas, K., Tonigan, J. S., Henry, M. C., Christian, K., Rodriguez, A., et al. (2021). Prenatal maternal posttraumatic stress disorder as a risk factor for adverse birth weight and gestational age outcomes: A systematic review and meta-analysis. *Journal of Affective Disorders, 295*, 530–540. https://doi.org/10.1016/j.jad.2021.08.079

Scott, K. A., Britton, L., & McLemore, M. R. (2019). The ethics of perinatal care for black women: Dismantling the structural racism in "mother blame" narratives. *The Journal of Perinatal & Neonatal Nursing, 33*(2), 108–115. https://doi.org/10.1097/JPN.0000000000000394

Seng, J., Miller, J., Sperlich, M., van de Ven, C. J., Brown, S., Carter, C. S., & Liberzon, I. (2013a). Exploring dissociation and oxytocin as pathways between trauma exposure and trauma-related hyperemesis gravidarum: A test-of-concept pilot. *Journal of Trauma & Dissociation, 14*(1), 40–55. https://doi.org/10.1080/15299732.2012.694594

Seng, J. S., Kohn-Wood, L. P., McPherson, M. D., & Sperlich, M. (2011). Disparity in posttraumatic stress disorder diagnosis among African American pregnant women. *Archives of Women's Mental Health, 14*(4), 295–306. https://doi.org/10.1007/s00737-011-0218-2

Seng, J. S., Li, Y., Yang, J. J., King, A. P., Low, L. M. K., Sperlich, M., et al. (2018). Gestational and postnatal cortisol profiles of women with posttraumatic stress disorder and the dissociative subtype. *Journal of Obstetric, Gynecologic & Neonatal Nursing, 47*(1), 12–22. https://doi.org/10.1016/j.jogn.2017.10.008

Seng, J. S., Low, L. M. K., Sperlich, M., Ronis, D. L., & Liberzon, I. (2009). Prevalence, trauma history, and risk for posttraumatic stress disorder among nulliparous women in maternity care. *Obstetrics and Gynecology, 114*(4), 839. https://doi.org/10.1097/AOG.0b013e3181b8f8a2

Seng, J. S., Sparbel, K. J., Low, L. K., & Killion, C. (2002). Abuse-related post-traumatic stress and desired maternity care practices: Women's perspectives. *Journal of Midwifery & Women's Health, 47*(5), 360–370. https://doi.org/10.1016/S1526-9523(02)00284-2

Seng, J. S., Sperlich, M., & Low, L. K. (2008). Mental health, demographic, and risk behavior profiles of pregnant survivors of childhood and adult abuse. *Journal of Midwifery & Women's Health, 53*(6), 511–521. https://doi.org/10.1016/j.jmwh.2008.04.013

Seng, J. S., Sperlich, M., Low, L. K., Ronis, D. L., Muzik, M., & Liberzon, I. (2013b). Childhood abuse history, posttraumatic stress disorder, postpartum mental health, and bonding: A prospective cohort study. *Journal of Midwifery & Women's Health, 58*(1), 57–68. https://doi.org/10.1111/j.1542-2011.2012.00237.x

Simkin, P., & Klaus, P. (2004). *When survivors give birth*. Classic Day.

Slade, P., Balling, K., Sheen, K., Goodfellow, L., Rymer, J., Spiby, H., & Weeks, A. (2020). Work-related post-traumatic stress symptoms in obstetricians and gynaecologists: Findings from INDIGO, a mixed-methods study with a cross-sectional survey and in-depth interviews. *BJOG: An International Journal of Obstetrics & Gynaecology, 127*(5), 600–608. https://doi.org/10.1111/1471-0528.16076

Sotero, M. (2006). A conceptual model of historical trauma: Implications for public health practice and research. *Journal of Health Disparities Research and Practice, 1*(1), 93–10. https://ssrn.com/abstract=1350062

Sperlich, M., & Seng, J. S. (2008). *Survivor moms: Women's stories of birthing, mothering and healing after sexual abuse*. Motherbaby Press.

Stein, D. J., Koenen, K. C., Friedman, M. J., Hill, E., McLaughlin, K. A., Petukhova, M., et al. (2013). Dissociation in posttraumatic stress disorder: Evidence from the world mental health surveys. *Biological Psychiatry, 73*(4), 302–312. https://doi.org/10.1016/j.biopsych.2012.08.022

Stein, M. B., McQuaid, J. R., Pedrelli, P., Lenox, R., & McCahill, M. E. (2000). Posttraumatic stress disorder in the primary care medical setting. *General Hospital Psychiatry, 22*(4), 261–269. https://doi.org/10.1016/S0163-8343(00)00080-3

Stevens, N. R., Miller, M. L., Puetz, A. K., Padin, A. C., Adams, N., & Meyer, D. J. (2021). Psychological intervention and treatment for posttraumatic stress disorder during pregnancy: A systematic review and call to action. *Journal of Traumatic Stress, 34*(3), 575–585. https://doi.org/10.1002/jts.22641

Teicher, M. H., Andersen, S. L., Polcari, A., Anderson, C. M., Navalta, C. P., & Kim, D. M. (2003). The neurobiological consequences of early stress and childhood maltreatment. *Neuroscience & Biobehavioral Reviews, 27*(1–2), 33–44. https://doi.org/10.1016/S0149-7634(03)00007-1

Van der Kolk, B. (2014). *The body keeps the score: Brain, mind, and body in the healing of trauma.* Penguin Press.

Weaver, I. C., Cervoni, N., Champagne, F. A., D'Alessio, A. C., Sharma, S., Seckl, J. R., et al. (2004). Epigenetic programming by maternal behavior. *Nature Neuroscience, 7*(8), 847–854. https://doi.org/10.1038/nn1276

Weinstein, A. D. (2016). *Prenatal development and parents' lived experiences: How early events shape our psychophysiology and relationships.* W. W. Norton & Company.

White, K. R., & Griffith, J. R. (2019). *The well-managed healthcare organization.* Health Administration Press.

World Health Organization. (2018). *ICD-11 for mortality and morbidity statistics.* https://icd.who.int/browse11/l-m/en

5

Childhood Abuse and Perinatal Depression, Anxiety, and Suicidal Thoughts and Behaviors

Cassandra Svelnys, Arianna Lane, and Angela J. Narayan ⓘ

Abstract Associations between childhood abuse and perinatal depression and anxiety are well documented, but less is known about the links between childhood abuse and perinatal suicidal thoughts and behaviors (STBs). This chapter applies a developmental psychopathology (DP) perspective to the pathways from childhood abuse to these three mental health problems and reviews key literature in three, brief sections. The first part includes an overview of theoretical pathways from childhood abuse to perinatal mental health problems according to the DP perspective and the concept of ghosts in the nursery. The second part describes several intervening mechanisms (e.g., emotion dysregulation, problems within social support networks, and disrupted stress biology) implicated in these pathways, including comorbidity of depression, anxiety, and STBs during the perinatal period, which itself may be a mechanism responsible for subsequent perinatal and postpartum outcomes. The third and final part of this

C. Svelnys • A. Lane • A. J. Narayan (✉)
Department of Psychology, University of Denver, Denver, CO, USA
e-mail: angela.narayan@du.edu

© The Author(s), under exclusive license to Springer Nature Switzerland AG 2023
R. Brunton, R. Dryer (eds.), *Perinatal Care and Considerations for Survivors of Child Abuse*, https://doi.org/10.1007/978-3-031-33639-3_5

chapter includes future directions focused on the need to improve the understanding of the effects of early life adversities and mental health problems in gender-diverse pregnant individuals, and to expand the focus to also characterize these pathways in biological or non-biological, non-gestational caregivers. The perinatal period is a window of opportunity when individuals more frequently access healthcare services, so clinical and practical efforts should capitalize on screening for and addressing the effects of unresolved childhood abuse, in addition to ongoing mental health problems, to intervene and promote resilience and well-being in parents, infants, and families as early in development as possible.

Keywords Childhood abuse • Depression • Anxiety • Suicidal thoughts and behavior • Developmental psychopathology • Ghosts in the nursery

The perinatal period is a major developmental experience characterized by a mixture of excitement, stress, vulnerability, and opportunity for many pregnant individuals (Davis & Narayan, 2020; Slade et al., 2009). In addition to the anticipation and hopefulness that comes with preparing to welcome a new baby, pregnancy can be a time of psychological upheaval, particularly for individuals with histories of childhood abuse (Narayan et al., 2017; Slade & Cohen, 1996; Sperlich & Seng, 2008). In thinking ahead and planning to care for a new baby, many individuals who were abused in childhood become haunted by negative or painful memories of these early adversities that they wish to avoid with their own children (Fraiberg et al., 1975; Narayan et al., 2019; Slade & Cohen, 1996).

In pregnant individuals, the rates of reported childhood abuse (e.g., emotional, physical, or sexual) range from 17% to more than 70%, with low-income, marginalized or minoritized individuals reporting the highest rates (Brunton & Dryer, 2021; Narayan et al., 2017; Seng et al., 2009). In this chapter, we use the term "pregnant individuals" to recognize that individuals with diverse gender identities, including (but not limited to) cisgender women, nonbinary individuals, and transgender men, may be capable of pregnancy, have the experience of becoming pregnant, and identify as a pregnant person (Moseson et al., 2021). Pregnancy and early postpartum are also periods when individuals are increasingly susceptible to mental health problems, including depression and anxiety symptoms, as well as elevated suicidal thoughts and behaviors (STBs), particularly if they have histories of childhood abuse (Atzl et al., 2019; Brunton & Dryer, 2021; Reid et al., 2022; Sperlich & Seng, 2008). Taken together, a history of childhood abuse and an increased risk of mental health problems during the perinatal period render many families particularly vulnerable to intergenerational maladaptation, including poorer individual perinatal adjustment, negative parent-infant relationships, and risks for abusive parenting in the next generation. As such, a thorough understanding of the pathways from childhood abuse to perinatal mental health problems is needed to inform efforts to prevent the transmission of trauma and psychopathology across generations and promote family resilience.

The purpose of this chapter is to provide a brief review of the literature on links between childhood abuse and mental health problems in individuals during the perinatal period (pregnancy through 12-months postpartum). While perinatal post-traumatic stress disorder (PTSD) is often a consequence of childhood abuse, as it reflects a sequelae of childhood trauma exposure to adulthood traumatic stress (Narayan et al., 2021; Seng et al., 2009), this review focuses on perinatal depression and anxiety, as these mental health issues are more common than PTSD (Davis & Narayan, 2020; Narayan et al., 2019), and PTSD has already been covered in Chap. 4.

We also focus on the links between childhood abuse and STBs in perinatal samples. This area is underdeveloped yet critical to understand due to the severe risk that STBs pose to parents' and infants' health, morbidity, and viability. For instance, suicide is a leading cause of death among pregnant and postpartum individuals (Shadigian & Bauer, 2005), and STBs are particularly elevated among pregnant individuals also experiencing depression (Lindahl et al., 2005). Furthermore, pregnant individuals may have a greater likelihood of experiencing STBs, such as suicidal ideation, than the general population, likely due to compounding mental health problems and relationship stressors that may accumulate during pregnancy (Gelaye et al., 2016; River et al., 2019). Perinatal STBs are also on the rise, according to recent evidence from a large U.S. study that revealed the prevalence of STBs during the perinatal period nearly tripled from 2006 to 2017 (Admon et al., 2021).

This chapter uses the developmental psychopathology (DP) perspective to succinctly review aspects of life-span pathways and intervening mechanisms from childhood abuse to perinatal depression, anxiety, and STBs. Part I applies the DP perspective to explain how childhood abuse may portend a risk of perinatal mental health problems. Part II covers several mechanisms (e.g., emotion dysregulation and a lack of effective coping skills, including STBs, problems within social support networks, and disrupted stress biology) linking childhood abuse to the specified mental health problems. Part III explains how these perinatal mental health problems are comorbid and transactional with each other, thereby becoming a mechanism that can propagate risk across generations. Part III then provides future directions and conclusions. Wherever possible, we focus our review on perinatal individuals with histories of childhood abuse specifically, as opposed to broader childhood adversity.

Part I: The Developmental Psychopathology (DP) Perspective and Intervening Mechanisms

The DP perspective theorizes that development is best understood as an integrative framework that considers how early experiences lay the foundation for later adaptation. Cumulative experiences and multi-system and multilevel factors also build on early experiences. Adaptation is characterized by the intersection of biological, psychological, and socio-contextual factors that influence both normative and atypical functioning across the life span (Cicchetti & Toth, 2009; Masten, 2006; Narayan et al., 2021; Sroufe, 2020).

The Developmental Psychopathology of Childhood Abuse

Several core principles of the DP perspective can be applied to the pathways linking childhood abuse to the specified perinatal mental health problems. According to the developmental principle of DP, deleterious early experiences, such as abuse, are particularly formative and enduring for subsequent adaptation and maladaptation (Narayan et al., 2021; Sroufe, 2020). Direct abuse of children is a particularly egregious developmental experience for several reasons. First, it may directly cause significant bodily harm. Second, if it is perpetrated by caregivers who would otherwise provide safety to children, it renders children helpless in the face of danger, leading to compounding risks of harm without protection (Cicchetti, 2016). Indeed, recent theoretical advances have suggested that childhood adversity, characterized specifically by threat (i.e., experiences characterized by physical harm to oneself or high potential of harm from violence in the environment, such as all three types of abuse covered here, as well as exposure to domestic or community violence), exerts robust effects on long-term development that are distinct from experiences of deprivation (i.e., inadequate access to basic needs or expected environmental inputs, such as any type of neglect, food or housing insecurity, or loss of a caregiver; Sheridan & McLaughlin, 2014). Therefore, childhood abuse, a large component of definitions of threat, may exert powerful and unique effects on long-term adaptation that are distinct from childhood neglect.

Maladaptive Development from Childhood to Pregnancy

A third consequence is that childhood abuse, in the form of emotional, physical, or sexual abuse, may impede or entirely prevent the normative development of emotion regulation skills. Infants' development of healthy emotion regulation heavily relies on sensitive and contingent responsiveness from caregivers, and on caregivers' scaffolding of infants' ability to co-regulate their emotional arousal and distress. Through these processes, children increasingly learn to cope independently with emotions (Sroufe, 2020; Thompson, 2019). When the caregiver(s) whom infants rely on for emotional safety and co-regulation are instead abusive or unable to protect children from abuse, infants not only cannot regulate and cope with their emotional arousal, but they may also experience intense emotional reactions characterized by fear or pain and a lack of ability to cope with this severe distress (Cicchetti, 2016; Lieberman et al., 2020; Sroufe, 2020).

Childhood abuse may interfere with the consolidation of healthy emotional identification, expression, and communication skills. For instance, abusive caregivers and caregiving environments may inhibit or invalidate young children's emotional displays (e.g., in the context of emotional abuse); respond punitively to children's emotional reactions, and model aggressive emotion regulation strategies (e.g., in the context of physical abuse); and, in extreme cases, directly elicit highly inappropriate and intense emotional and physiological arousal (e.g., in the context of sexual abuse), all of which are extremely harmful to subsequent development (Brunton & Dryer, 2021; Cicchetti, 2016; Lieberman et al., 2020; Sperlich & Seng, 2008). Abusive caregivers, in turn, may evoke children's fear or avoidance of caregivers, rather than help children to develop healthy and effective emotion regulation and coping skills (Sroufe, 2020; Thompson, 2019). Lacking adequate opportunities for healthy emotional development to be consolidated, abused individuals may enter adulthood and pregnancy with poor emotion identification, regulation, and coping skills. This may become particularly problematic when individuals face stressors inherent to pregnancy (e.g., hormonal, physiological and physical changes, negotiation and division of caregiving roles with a co-parent, and unexpected pregnancy-related complications or concerns).

Ghosts in the Nursery

When they become pregnant and experience stress, adults with abuse histories may experience intense emotional flooding, without resources to engage in healthy coping strategies. Fraiberg and colleagues' seminal "ghosts in the nursery" metaphor highlights that for adults with a history of childhood abuse, several aspects of the perinatal experience may serve as trauma reminders for unresolved childhood abuse and awaken long-forgotten negative memories and feelings (Fraiberg et al., 1975; Narayan et al., 2016). According to this theory, a developing child often does not consciously retain the intense emotional anguish (e.g., fear, pain, anger) associated with abuse from their caregivers because this poses a fundamental psychological dilemma: *My caregiver who is supposed to be protecting and loving me is instead hurting or violating me.* This dilemma is unbearable for a young child, who, in turn, disengages from this anguish and often only consciously remembers the physical acts of abuse themselves in the absence of the pain they caused (Fraiberg et al., 1975; Lieberman et al., 2020).

When abused children become adults, these abusive behaviors become their caregiving templates and are most likely to be used when young offspring display undesirable emotions and behaviors (e.g., fussing, screaming, acting out). Many of these undesirable behaviors are normative child responses that signal needs or discomfort (e.g., crying because of hunger or fatigue) or serve as bids for physical contact or co-regulation. However, parents with abuse histories may incorrectly interpret them as negative intentions to consciously displease the parent. For instance, an infant's loud or unrelenting crying from being hungry, needing their diaper changed, or wanting to be picked up may serve as a trauma reminder for the parent's own unresolved anguish, which is the ghost in the nursery that continues to haunt the parent. The parent's internalized template of caregiving may predominantly include abusive responses that they experienced when crying as a small child (e.g., being hit, yelled at, or told to "shut up"). The parent may then respond abusively by reenacting their internalized template with infants that, in turn, perpetrates the intergenerational transmission of abusive caregiving (Fraiberg et al., 1975; Lieberman et al., 2005).

Other trauma reminders that may haunt abused pregnant individuals may also include the unexpected physiological or bodily in-utero sensations related to fetal development or unwanted or unexpected physical interventions during labor (e.g., a provider checking the individual's cervix, rotating the baby in the birth canal, or using forceps or vacuum extraction during delivery) to facilitate labor. These experiences may remind pregnant individuals of physical harm or bodily violation that they suffered as children and may, in turn, trigger severe emotional dysregulation, dissociation, anger, and traumatic stress, in addition to parent-child attachment problems and lower perceived parenting competence

(Berthelot et al., 2019a; Berthelot et al., 2019b; Fraiberg et al., 1975; Lieberman et al., 2020; Narayan et al., 2016; Slade & Cohen, 1996).

In addition to present-moment psychological distress during the perinatal period, labor, and delivery, and in the early postpartum period, ghosts in the nursery would be expected to increase or exacerbate perinatal depression, anxiety, and, in extreme cases, STBs. For instance, many caregivers with childhood abuse histories are insightfully aware that they do not want to repeat the same abusive acts of their parents. However, they are not aware of alternative, positive parenting strategies to use instead. This understandable lack of knowledge, combined with ongoing trauma reminders of their abusive past elicited during periods of heightened infant distress, may contribute to depression, anxiety, and hopelessness. While becoming aware of the harmful effects of one's own abuse is often the first step in breaking intergenerational cycles of abusive caregiving, many pregnant or postpartum individuals may feel at a loss about effective parenting strategies to use instead and may experience emotional dysregulation and despair if supportive interventions or parenting resources are not accessible to them (Lieberman et al., 2020; Narayan et al., 2016; Sperlich & Seng, 2008).

Part II: Mechanisms Linking Child Abuse to Perinatal Depression, Anxiety, and STBs

This section continues to draw upon the DP perspective and review empirical findings on intervening mechanisms linking childhood abuse and perinatal depression, anxiety, and STBs. We continue to apply several specific DP principles to pathways of childhood abuse to perinatal mental health problems. All DP principles are also detailed in Table 5.1 with relevant examples.

Emotion Dysregulation

As children progress through early and middle childhood, healthy social adaptation requires children to strengthen coping skills and

Table 5.1 Developmental psychopathology principles and examples

Principle	Definition	Example 1: Childhood abuse	Example 2: Perinatal depression, anxiety, and STBs
Developmental principle	Early life influences (e.g., experiences, relationships, environmental factors) are enduring and formative for developmental health and adaptation.[1,2]	Childhood abuse (e.g., emotional/verbal, physical, and sexual) may have long-lasting effects on adulthood and perinatal functioning via compromising emotional regulation, stress reactivity, and expectations about safety in relationships.[5,6]	Individuals with childhood physical abuse may have caregiving templates of abusive parenting practices. The desire to parent differently but a lack of positive alternatives may increase the risk of prenatal and postpartum depression, anxiety, and STBs, especially when infants are distressed.[12,14]
Agency principle	Individuals play an active role in their development, simultaneously influencing and being influenced by their relationships, experiences, and contexts.[1,3]	Children who are abused may engage in physical or verbal aggression with peers or romantic partners to protect themselves, potentially eliciting further aggression from social counterparts.[4,7]	Individuals with childhood abuse histories may respond to perinatal interpersonal conflict by being verbally or physically aggressive, which, in turn, may compromise relationship support, amplify conflict, and increase isolation, depression symptoms, and STBs.[7,8]

(continued)

Table 5.1 (continued)

Principle	Definition	Example 1: Childhood abuse	Example 2: Perinatal depression, anxiety, and STBs
Normative/ mutually informative principle	The emergence of mental health problems is best understood while also considering pathways of healthy, competent functioning. One must understand how development typically progresses to understand how psychopathology emerges.[4]	While all children struggle with emotion regulation skills at times, abused children may more frequently experience negative emotions (e.g., fear, anger, sadness) while also lacking safe and consistent caregivers to help them co-regulate and cope with negative emotions.[5,6]	Individuals from cultures that view physical discipline as socially normative may appraise their childhood experiences differently than individuals raised in cultures that do not use physical discipline. Cultural match of perinatal care providers with perinatal individuals' cultural backgrounds decreases stigma, depression, and anxiety during pregnancy.[13,15]
Systems principle	Individuals are embedded within interacting systems at the level of families, communities, and societies. Development is shaped by dynamic interplay between all nested systems.[1,3]	Pregnant individuals with histories of childhood abuse perpetrated by a caregiver may be less likely to rely on that caregiver for support during pregnancy, thereby restricting their support system.[8]	Restricted social support from caregivers may contribute to perinatal depression and STBs, as well as isolation and withdrawal, which in turn, may interfere with accessing other social support.[7,8]

(continued)

Table 5.1 (continued)

Principle	Definition	Example 1: Childhood abuse	Example 2: Perinatal depression, anxiety, and STBs
Multilevel principle	Development proceeds at multiple levels of functioning (e.g., biological, physiological, cognitive, emotional, behavioral), so multiple levels of analysis are needed to understand pathways of typical versus atypical development.[3,5]	Childhood abuse affects multiple levels of development, including neurobiological, cognitive, and psychological functioning; stress reactivity; emotional regulation; and behavioral responses.[5,7]	A history of unresolved childhood abuse may influence mental health problems and alterations in stress physiology during pregnancy, and lead to dysregulation of stress biology across generations.[11,13]
Equifinality principle	Many different developmental experiences may converge on similar pathways or outcomes.[1,2,3]	Many different types of childhood abuse (e.g., emotional, physical, or sexual) may confer risk for depression, anxiety, and STBs across adolescence or adulthood.[9,10]	Pregnant individuals' STBs may stem from several influences, including reminders of childhood abuse, ongoing life stressors, or intimate partner violence victimization during pregnancy.[9,12,13]

(continued)

Table 5.1 (continued)

Principle	Definition	Example 1: Childhood abuse	Example 2: Perinatal depression, anxiety, and STBs
Multifinality principle	One set of developmental experiences may lead to a variety of different outcomes within or across individuals.[3,5]	For some individuals, childhood abuse is associated with greater HPA-axis dysregulation during pregnancy, such as elevated cortisol awakening responses and higher-than-typical cortisol concentrations. Other abused individuals display blunted cortisol responses and lower-than-typical concentrations during pregnancy.[11]	Following childhood abuse, maladaptive alterations in physiological functioning across development may render pregnant individuals more vulnerable to many mental health problems, such as anxiety, depression, STBs, and various comorbidities.[11,13]

(*continued*)

Table 5.1 (continued)

Principle	Definition	Example 1: Childhood abuse	Example 2: Perinatal depression, anxiety, and STBs
Longitudinal principle	Development does not have a singular endpoint because early life, cumulative, and contemporaneous experiences shape adaptation and maladaptation across the life span and over generations.[3,4]	The long-term effects of childhood abuse may lead to difficulties with emotion regulation and increased distress in reflecting on one's childhood, both during pregnancy and parenthood.[2,6,12]	Individuals with childhood abuse histories are at risk for depression, anxiety, and STBs across development and during pregnancy, and their children are also at higher risk for abusive caregiving and mental health problems.[2,9,13]
Resilience principle	Resilience is defined as successful adaptation by an individual or system during or following adversity to promote survival, viability, and functioning.[2,3]	Many individuals with histories of childhood abuse do not go on to experience perinatal mental health problems, and most abused individuals do not have children who are abused.[2]	Social support from family, friends, and healthcare providers in addition to the romantic partner or co-parent is a key protective factor against the effects of childhood abuse on perinatal depression, anxiety, and STBs.[2,8,15]

Note. 1. Cicchetti and Toth (2009), 2. Narayan et al. (2021), 3. Masten (2006), 4. Sroufe (2020), 5. Cicchetti (2016), 6. Heleniak et al. (2016), 7. River et al. (2019), 8. Atzl et al. (2019), 9. Yates et al. (2008), 10. Brunton and Dryer (2021), 11. Davis and Narayan (2020), 12. Slade et al. (2009), 13. Sperlich and Seng (2008), 14. Lieberman et al. (2005), 15. Narayan et al. (2016).

independently identify and apply a range of possible emotional responses to different interpersonal interactions (Sroufe, 2020; Thompson, 2019). As such, children increasingly implement coping strategies to manage emotional, physiological, and behavioral responses to social situations (Boldt et al., 2020). Consistent with the developmental and systems principles of DP that assume experiences build across development and transact across social systems, abused children may learn to disengage from their emotions and avoid emotional reactions, resulting in possible hypoactivity (e.g., under-responding, emotional suppression) in response to both positive and negative social interactions (Cicchetti, 2016). This emotional hypoactivity may be characterized by maladaptive patterns of internal emotion processing (e.g., elevated depression symptoms or anger rumination) and missed opportunities to hone adaptive emotion regulation skills with help from social counterparts, such as friends or teachers (Heleniak et al., 2016; Lavi et al., 2019; Sroufe, 2020; Thompson, 2019; Zhu et al., 2020). As an alternate possibility, abused children may also show biases toward more quickly recognizing negative emotions and less quickly recognizing positive emotions, resulting in tendencies to overreact to neutral or ambiguous social interactions with angry or aggressive responses (Pollak et al., 2000; Zhu et al., 2020).

Across development and into adulthood, patterns of emotion dysregulation among individuals with histories of abuse may include difficulties controlling the intensity and duration of emotional responses; incongruence of emotional response to context; tendencies to react with anger, aggression, and impulsivity; and rumination of negative emotions (Heleniak et al., 2016; Lavi et al., 2019). Specifically, in the perinatal period, one study found that emotion dysregulation mediated the path from a history of childhood abuse to negative emotionality (i.e., a composite of anxiety, depression, and stress symptoms) during pregnancy (Greene et al., 2021). Pregnant individuals with experiences of unresolved childhood abuse may also harbor intense negative feelings, including self-criticism, lack adequate coping strategies to respond to pregnancy-related stressors, suppress difficult emotions, and display impulsive emotional responses, such as angry outbursts and self-injurious behaviors (Sperlich & Seng, 2008). All these difficulties may exacerbate the risk of perinatal anxiety, depression, and

STBs and increase the risk of parental-fetal stress transmission (Buss et al., 2017; Davis & Narayan, 2020).

Maladaptive Coping Skills

According to the life-span principle of DP, development does not have an endpoint, and the effects of harmful early experiences such as abuse may have enduring effects into adulthood and across generations (Masten, 2006; Narayan et al., 2021). Children exposed to abusive and threatening responses to their emotions may continue to engage in emotion suppression or avoidance patterns through adulthood. When a pregnant person with a history of child abuse prepares to engage in parenting themself, they may lack adequate coping skills to manage intense and unexpected stress due to shifting moods, fluctuating hormones, and increased daily demands (e.g., prenatal appointments, preparation to take leave from work, accrual of baby supplies). These stressors, combined with preexisting deficits in recruiting effective emotion regulation skills, may become potent risk factors for STBs during pregnancy (Reid et al., 2022; Yates et al., 2008). High levels of prenatal distress and failure to cope may lead to unwanted or intrusive suicidal thoughts and, potentially, self-injurious behaviors and substance use, particularly for individuals who have resorted to self-harm behaviors in the past (Gelaye et al., 2016; Sperlich & Seng, 2008).

Problems Within Social Support Networks

The systems and multilevel principles of DP apply to the pathways from childhood abuse to interpersonal functioning in pregnant individuals. These principles delineate that individuals are nested within their broader interpersonal networks of social interactions and that development consolidates as the result of processes across multiple levels of functioning (e.g., biological, physiological, cognitive, emotional, behavioral; Masten, 2006; Cicchetti, 2016). In terms of the systems principle, the presence of childhood abuse and the absence of adulthood social support are two strong and often related predictors of prenatal depression and anxiety symptoms (Biaggi et al., 2016). For instance, abuse perpetrated by a childhood caregiver may, in turn, prevent a pregnant individual from utilizing this caregiver for emotional, psychological, or material support during the perinatal period, thereby limiting their support system (Atzl et al., 2019; Easterbrooks et al., 2011). Additionally, individuals who experienced childhood abuse may have poorer social relationships with romantic partners, friends, or other sources of support (Narayan et al., 2021; Sroufe, 2020). Indeed, poorer relationship quality, including lower levels of support from and higher levels of conflict with the other biological parent, has been found to fully mediate the association between childhood abuse and depression symptoms during pregnancy (River et al., 2019). Alternatively, social support from other individuals (e.g., family, friends, healthcare providers), in addition to pregnant individuals' romantic partner or co-parent, has been identified as a key protective factor against perinatal depression, anxiety, and STBs (Atzl et al., 2019; Gelaye et al., 2016; River et al., 2019). These findings underscore that the adjustment and well-being of pregnant individuals are nested within their social context and can shield them against perinatal mental health problems and the transmission of abuse and psychopathology across generations (Lieberman et al., 2020).

Disrupted Stress Biology

Consistent with the multilevel principle of DP, childhood abuse has been associated with disruptions to normative stress responses at the biological level, such as dysregulation of the hypothalamic-pituitary-adrenal (HPA) axis (Bowers & Yehuda, 2016; Davis & Narayan, 2020). Changes in stress physiology are part of normative processes during pregnancy, which include the secretion of corticotropin-releasing hormone (CRH) by the hypothalamus and the fetal placenta, as well as a decrease in parental HPA-axis responsivity to stress (Davis & Narayan, 2020). However, dysregulation of the HPA-axis, including both hyperactivity and hypoactivity, has been suggested to adversely affect the parent and child (Bowers & Yehuda, 2016). For instance, some pregnant individuals with abuse histories experience elevated cortisol awakening responses and prolonged, higher-than-typical concentrations of cortisol during pregnancy (hypercortisolemia), while other pregnant individuals have lower levels of cortisol than needed (hypocortisolemia; Buss et al., 2017; Scheyer & Urizar Jr., 2016; Schreier et al., 2015; Seth et al., 2016).

Similarly, for some individuals who experienced child abuse, it may be adaptive for their stress response symptoms to show blunted physiological arousal to threat to reduce wear on the body and regulatory systems associated with chronic activation of stress responses. However, hypoactivity of stress response to subsequent stressors, specifically stressful experiences more proximal to pregnancy (e.g., conflict with co-parent, sleep difficulties), may result in poorer coping with contemporaneous daily challenges (e.g., managing work and income, taking care of other children, navigating physical illness or pain) and increase the risk of prenatal mental health problems (Bowers & Yehuda, 2016; Reid et al., 2022). Furthermore, both hypercortisolemia and hypocortisolemia are linked to a heightened risk of developing postnatal depressive symptoms, although each may predict a unique symptom profile. For instance, hypercortisolemia may be associated with a more temporary or intermittent depressed mood, whereas hypocortisolemia may be associated with more stable and chronic postpartum depression (Seth et al., 2016). Additionally, individual differences in cortisol regulation, characteristics of the childhood abuse (e.g., developmental timing, intensity, frequency, chronicity, and identity of the perpetrator), and historical and ongoing mental health problems likely influence and complicate these patterns (Bowers & Yehuda, 2016; Buss et al., 2017; Davis & Narayan, 2020).

Furthermore, although beyond the scope of the review, adulthood sleep disturbance is another likely intervening mechanism implicated in the pathway between childhood abuse and perinatal mental health (Fuligni et al., 2021). For example, recent findings demonstrated that childhood maltreatment specifically, as opposed to childhood adversity within the family more broadly, predicted pregnant individuals' sleep quality even after accounting for current stressors during pregnancy (Nevarez-Brewster et al., 2022). Understanding patterns and pathways from childhood abuse to dysregulated stress physiology and other biological systems (e.g., sleep, as well as nutritional and cardiometabolic systems) during the perinatal period are emerging research areas with implications for understanding the risk of depression, anxiety, and STBs.

Part III: Comorbidities and Conclusions

Perinatal depression and anxiety are highly comorbid during the perinatal period (Davis & Narayan, 2020). In childbearing individuals, an estimated 9.5% and 8.2%, respectively, report comorbid depressive and anxiety symptomatology prenatally and postnatally (Falah-Hassani et al., 2017). Perinatal depression and anxiety also co-occur with STBs, particularly for individuals with a history of childhood abuse (Sperlich & Seng, 2008). Thus, comorbid mental health problems and their transactional effects with other mechanistic influences (e.g., comorbid mental health problems interfering with adaptive stress physiology, coping skills, and quality of social support) may themselves become a mechanism amplifying effects of childhood abuse on labor, delivery, birth, and infant outcomes (discussed more in Chap. 5).

Comorbidity of Perinatal Mental Health Problems

Given that research has found that childhood abuse predicts both prenatal anxiety and depression on their own (Biaggi et al., 2016) and that prenatal anxiety and depression are often comorbid (Davis & Narayan, 2020), it stands to reason that childhood abuse may also increase the risk of co-occurring perinatal depression, anxiety, and STBs during the perinatal period. Among individuals with perinatal depression, approximately one-third also report suicidal ideation during pregnancy (Mauri et al., 2012). Furthermore, in a cohort of pregnant individuals referred to a mental health unit in the U.K. for previous postpartum depression, 24% endorsed a suicide attempt during a prior postnatal period of a previous pregnancy (Healey et al., 2013). Although Healey and colleagues did not report what proportion of these expecting parents had histories of childhood abuse, another study found that the effects of childhood abuse and current depression appear to be additive—pregnant individuals with both risk factors have greater odds of experiencing suicidal ideation than those with neither risk factor (Chin et al., 2022).

Evidence also indicates that experiences of childhood abuse, and particularly physical abuse, are linked to perinatal STBs (Reid et al., 2022), which are also more prevalent among those with comorbid perinatal depression or anxiety (Gelaye et al., 2016). Furthermore, though perinatal anxiety, depression, and STBs are separately associated with health complications for the pregnant individual and the fetus, comorbid anxiety and depression, particularly in individuals with histories of childhood abuse, may portend an even greater risk of infants' negative outcomes, such as premature birth, low birth weight, increased cortisol production, reduced maternal-infant bonding, sleep disturbances, and infant neurological impairment (Choi, 2018; Deutsch et al., 2022; Evans et al., 2008; Field et al., 2010). Overall, research on comorbid perinatal mental health problems, including depression, anxiety, and STBs, specifically in individuals with a history of childhood abuse, continues to be underdeveloped, so future research should clarify the prevalence and impact of these comorbidities on this vulnerable population.

Future Directions and Conclusions

Research on pathways by which childhood abuse affects perinatal anxiety, depression, and STBs has increased in recent years, with greater utilization of longitudinal studies and inclusion of mechanisms (e.g., emotion regulation, coping ability, social support, stress biology) implicated across childhood development to the pregnancy and postpartum periods. Additionally, recent studies have begun to consider how socio-contextual factors (e.g., race, ethnicity, socioeconomic status) may influence pathways from childhood abuse to perinatal well-being, especially among individuals with minoritized and marginalized identities (Narayan et al., 2019). However, there are still notable gaps in these areas, and several important avenues remain largely understudied. Consideration of perinatal STBs has increased, yet underlying mechanisms from childhood abuse to the development and maintenance of STBs require further investigation to inform intervention efforts. Additionally, most longitudinal studies of childhood adversity to perinatal outcomes focus on pregnancies resulting in a live birth, while less research has examined factors associated with the termination of pregnancy (e.g., miscarriage, abortion) or early mortem (e.g., fetal and infant death) in individuals with histories of childhood abuse, let alone how a history of childhood abuse as well as perinatal mental health problems may be associated with reproductive or fertility problems.

Furthermore, the vast majority of research on the perinatal period has been limited to the experiences of cisgender, heterosexual women. Gender-diverse individuals experience an increased risk of childhood abuse and unintended pregnancy (Alley et al., 2022; Tobin & Delaney, 2019), yet virtually no research exists examining pathways from childhood abuse to perinatal depression, anxiety, and STBs among these individuals. There is a notable scarcity of perinatal research that considers the experiences of LGBTQ+ pregnant individuals and non-gestational partners. Furthermore, pathways between childhood abuse and perinatal mental health problems in either biological or non-biological, non-gestational parents (i.e., biological fathers, gender-diverse co-parents) have only recently been included in perinatal research (e.g., Narayan et al., 2019). The inclusion of non-gestational parents in perinatal research needs to be prioritized, given the potential for important biological influences (e.g., during fertilization), relationship dynamics (e.g., co-parenting conflict versus support), and psychological contributions (e.g., the second parents' mental health) that affect parental, fetal, and infant development.

In conclusion, the perinatal period is a time of increased hope and optimism for many families, yet it may also represent a period of increased vulnerability to perinatal depression, anxiety, and STBs for individuals with histories of childhood abuse. The complex and transactional psychological, biological, and social changes that occur during this transformative time underscore the perinatal period as an important window for preventive intervention to address and decrease unresolved childhood abuse, ghosts in the nursery, and mental health symptoms. During pregnancy, individuals often receive more frequent and predictable medical care, so perinatal health service appointments may be opportunities to screen for the effects of unresolved childhood abuse, discussed more in Chap. 7 of this volume, in addition to the risk of depression, anxiety, and STBS. More comprehensive knowledge of the experiences of diverse pregnant individuals is especially needed, as are inclusive perinatal services, resources, and interventions for all caregivers, gestational or otherwise, to reduce the effects of childhood abuse and mental health problems and promote families' intergenerational resilience.

References

Admon, L. K., Dalton, V. K., Kolenic, G. E., Ettner, S. L., Tilea, A., Haffajee, R. L., Brownlee, R. M., Zochowski, M. K., Tabb, K. M., Muzik, M., & Zivin, K. (2021). Trends in suicidality 1 year before and after birth among commercially-insured childbearing individuals in the United States, 2006–2017. *JAMA Psychiatry, 78*, 171–176. https://doi.org/10.1001/jamapsychiatry.2020.3550

Alley, J., Jenkins, V., Everett, B., & Diamond, L. M. (2022). Understanding the link between adolescent same-gender contact and unintended pregnancy: The role of early adversity and sexual risk behavior. *Archives of Sexual Behavior, 51*, 1839–1855. https://doi.org/10.1007/s10508-021-02143-0

Atzl, V. M., Grande, L. A., Davis, E. P., & Narayan, A. J. (2019). Perinatal promotive and protective factors for women with histories of childhood abuse and neglect. *Child Abuse & Neglect, 91*, 63–77. https://doi.org/10.1016/j.chiabu.2019.02.008

Berthelot, N., Lemieux, R., Garon-Bissonnette, J., Lacharité, C., & Muzik, M. (2019a). The protective role of mentalizing: Reflective functioning as a mediator between child maltreatment, psychopathology and parental attitude in expecting parents. *Child Abuse & Neglect, 95*, 104065. https://doi.org/10.1016/j.chiabu.2019.104065

Berthelot, N., Lemieux, R., Garon-Bissonnette, J., & Muzik, M. (2019b). Prenatal attachment, parental confidence, and mental health in expecting parents: The role of childhood trauma. *Journal of Midwifery & Women's Health, 65*, 85–95. https://doi.org/10.1111/jmwh.13034

Biaggi, A., Conroy, S., Pawlby, S., & Pariante, C. M. (2016). Identifying the women at risk of antenatal anxiety and depression: A systematic review. *Journal of Affective Disorders, 191*, 62–77. https://doi.org/10.1016/j.jad.2015.11.014

Boldt, L. J., Goffin, K. C., & Kochanska, G. (2020). The significance of early parent-child attachment for emerging regulation: A longitudinal investigation of processes and mechanisms from toddler age to preadolescence. *Developmental Psychology, 56*, 431–443. https://doi.org/10.1037/dev0000862

Bowers, M. E., & Yehuda, R. (2016). Intergenerational transmission of stress in humans. *Neuropsychopharmacology, 41*, 232–244. https://doi.org/10.1038/npp.2015.247

Brunton, R., & Dryer, R. (2021). Child sexual abuse and pregnancy: A systematic review of the literature. *Child Abuse & Neglect, 111*, 104802. https://doi.org/10.1016/j.chiabu.2020.104802

Buss, C., Entringer, S., Moog, N. K., Toepfer, P., Fair, D. A., Simhan, H. N., Heim, C. M., & Wadhwa, P. D. (2017). Intergenerational transmission of maternal childhood maltreatment exposure: Implications for fetal brain development. *Journal of the American Academy of Child and Adolescent Psychiatry, 56*, 373–382. https://doi.org/10.1016/j.jaac.2017.03.001

Chin, K., Wendt, A., Bennett, I. M., & Bhat, A. (2022). Suicide and maternal mortality. *Current Psychiatry Reports, 24*(4), 239–275. https://doi.org/10.1007/s11920-022-01334-3

Choi, K. W. (2018). *Postpartum depression in the intergenerational transmission of child maltreatment: Longitudinal evidence from global settings.* Dissertation Abstracts International: Section B: The Sciences and Engineering, 78(12-B(E)).

Cicchetti, D. (2016). Socioemotional, personality, and biological development: Illustrations from a multilevel developmental psychopathology perspective on child maltreatment. *Annual Review of Psychology, 67*, 187–211. https://doi.org/10.1146/annurev-psych-122414-033259

Cicchetti, D., & Toth, S. L. (2009). The past achievements and future promises of developmental psychopathology: The coming of age of a discipline. *Journal of Child Psychology and Psychiatry, and Allied Disciplines, 50*, 16–25. https://doi.org/10.1111/j.1469-7610.2008.01979.x

Davis, E. P., & Narayan, A. J. (2020). Pregnancy as a period of risk, adaptation, and resilience for mothers and infants. *Development and Psychopathology, 32*, 1625–1639. https://doi.org/10.1017/S0954579420001121

Deutsch, A. R., Vargas, M. C., Lucchini, M., Brink, L. T., Odendaal, H. J., & Elliott, A. J. (2022). Effect of individual or comorbid antenatal depression and anxiety on birth outcomes and moderation by maternal traumatic experiences and resilience. *Journal of Affective Disorders Reports, 9*, 100365. https://doi.org/10.1016/j.jadr.2022.100365

Easterbrooks, M. A., Chaudhuri, J. H., Bartlett, J. D., & Copeman, A. (2011). Resilience in parenting among young mothers: Family and ecological risks and opportunities. *Children and Youth Services Review, 33*, 42–50. https://doi.org/10.1016/j.childyouth.2010.08.010

Evans, L. M., Myers, M. M., & Monk, C. (2008). Pregnant women's cortisol is elevated with anxiety and depression - but only when comorbid. *Archives of Women's Mental Health, 11*, 239–248. https://doi.org/10.1007/s00737-008-0019-4

Falah-Hassani, K., Shiri, R., & Dennis, C. L. (2017). The prevalence of antenatal and postnatal co-morbid anxiety and depression: A meta-analysis. *Psychological Medicine, 47*, 2041–2053. https://doi.org/10.1017/S0033291717000617

Field, T., Diego, M., Hernandez-Reif, M., Figueiredo, B., Deeds, O., Ascencio, A., Schanberg, S., & Kuhn, C. (2010). Comorbid depression and anxiety effects on pregnancy and neonatal outcome. *Infant Behavior and Development, 33*, 23–29. https://doi.org/10.1016/j.infbeh.2009.10.004

Fraiberg, S., Adelson, E., & Shapiro, V. (1975). Ghosts in the nursery. *Journal of the American Academy of Child Psychiatry, 14*(3), 387–421. https://doi.org/10.1016/S0002-7138(09)61442-4

Fuligni, A. J., Chiang, J. J., & Tottenham, N. (2021). Sleep disturbance and the long-term impact of early adversity. *Neuroscience & Biobehavioral Reviews, 126*, 304–313. https://doi.org/10.1016/j.neubiorev.2021.03.021

Gelaye, B., Kajeepeta, S., & Williams, M. A. (2016). Suicidal ideation in pregnancy: An epidemiologic review. *Archives of Women's Mental Health, 19*, 741–751. https://doi.org/10.1007/s00737-016-0646-0

Greene, C. A., McCoach, D. B., Briggs-Gowan, M. J., & Grasso, D. J. (2021). Associations among childhood threat and deprivation experiences, emotion dysregulation, and mental health in pregnant women. *Psychological Trauma: Theory, Research, Practice and Policy, 13*, 446–456. https://doi.org/10.1037/tra0001013

Healey, C., Morriss, R., Henshaw, C., Wadoo, O., Sajjad, A., Scholefield, H., & Kinderman, P. (2013). Self-harm in postpartum depression and referrals to a perinatal mental health team: An audit study. *Archives of Women's Mental Health, 16*, 237–245. https://doi.org/10.1007/s00737-013-0335-1

Heleniak, C., Jenness, J. L., Vander Stoep, A., McCauley, E., & McLaughlin, K. A. (2016). Childhood maltreatment exposure and disruptions in emotion regulation: A transdiagnostic pathway to adolescent internalizing and externalizing psychopathology. *Cognitive Therapy and Research, 40*, 394–415. https://doi.org/10.1007/s10608-015-9735-z

Lavi, I., Katz, L. F., Ozer, E. J., & Gross, J. J. (2019). Emotion reactivity and regulation in maltreated children: A meta-analysis. *Child Development, 90*, 1503–1524. https://doi.org/10.1111/cdev.13272

Lieberman, A. F., Diaz, M., Castro, G., & Oliver Bucio, G. (2020). *Make room for baby: Perinatal Child-Parent Psychotherapy to repair trauma and promote attachment.* Guilford Press.

Lieberman, A. F., Padrón, E., Van Horn, P., & Harris, W. W. (2005). Angels in the nursery: The intergenerational transmission of benevolent parental influences. *Infant Mental Health Journal, 26*, 504–520. https://doi.org/10.1002/imhj.20071

Lindahl, V., Pearson, J. L., & Colpe, L. (2005). Prevalence of suicidality during pregnancy and the postpartum. *Archives of Women's Mental Health, 8*, 77–87. https://doi.org/10.1007/s00737-005-0080-1

Masten, A. S. (2006). Developmental psychopathology: Pathways to the future. *International Journal of Behavioral Development, 30*, 47–54. https://doi.org/10.1177/0165025406059974

Mauri, M., Oppo, A., Borri, C., Banti, S., & PND-ReScU group. (2012). Suicidality in the perinatal period: Comparison of two self-report instruments. Results from PND-ReScU. *Archives of Women's Mental Health, 15*, 39–47. https://doi.org/10.1007/s00737-011-0246-y

Moseson, H., Fix, L., Hastings, J., Stoeffler, A., Lunn, M. R., Flentje, A., Lubensky, M. E., Capriotti, M. R., Ragosta, S., Forsberg, H., & Obedin-Maliver, J. (2021). Pregnancy intentions and outcomes among transgender, nonbinary, and gender-expansive people assigned female or intersex at birth in the United States: Results from a national, quantitative survey. *International Journal of Transgender Health, 22*, 30–41. https://doi.org/10.1080/2689526 9.2020.1841058

Narayan, A. J., Atzl, V. M., Merrick, J. S., River, L. M., & Pena, R. (2019). Therapeutic perinatal research with low-income families. *Zero to Three, 39*, 43–53.

Narayan, A. J., Lieberman, A. F., & Masten, A. S. (2021). Intergenerational transmission and prevention of adverse childhood experiences (ACEs). *Clinical Psychology Review, 85*, 101997. https://doi.org/10.1016/j.cpr.2021.101997

Narayan, A. J., Oliver Bucio, G., Rivera, L. M., & Lieberman, A. F. (2016). Making sense of the past creates space for the baby: Perinatal child-parent psychotherapy for pregnant women with childhood trauma. *Zero to Three, 36*, 22–28.

Narayan, A. J., Rivera, L. M., Bernstein, R. E., Castro, G., Gantt, T., Thomas, M., Nau, M., Harris, W. W., & Lieberman, A. F. (2017). Between pregnancy and motherhood: Identifying unmet mental health needs in pregnant women with lifetime adversity. *Zero to Three, 37*, 4–13.

Nevarez-Brewster, M., Aran, Ö., Narayan, A. J., Harrall, K. K., Brown, S. M., Hankin, B. L., & Davis, E. P. (2022). Adverse and benevolent childhood experiences predict prenatal sleep quality. *Adversity and Resilience Science, 1–12*, 391. https://doi.org/10.1007/s42844-022-00070-0

Pollak, S. D., Cicchetti, D., Hornung, K., & Reed, A. (2000). Recognizing emotion in faces: Developmental effects of child abuse and neglect. *Developmental Psychology, 36*, 679–688. https://doi.org/10.1037/0012-1649.36.5.679

Reid, H. E., Pratt, D., Edge, D., & Wittkowski, A. (2022). Maternal suicide ideation and behaviour during pregnancy and the first postpartum year: A systematic review of psychological and psychosocial risk factors. *Frontiers in Psychiatry, 13*, 765118. https://doi.org/10.3389/fpsyt.2022.765118

River, L. M., Narayan, A. J., Atzl, V. M., Rivera, L. M., & Lieberman, A. F. (2019). Past made present: The legacy of childhood maltreatment for romantic relationship quality and psychopathology during pregnancy. *Psychology of Violence, 10*, 324–333. https://doi.org/10.1037/vio0000273

Scheyer, K., & Urizar, G. G., Jr. (2016). Altered stress patterns and increased risk for postpartum depression among low-income pregnant women. *Archives of Women's Mental Health, 19*(2), 317–328. https://doi.org/10.1007/s00737-015-0563-7

Schreier, H. M., Enlow, M. B., Ritz, T., Gennings, C., & Wright, R. J. (2015). Childhood abuse is associated with increased hair cortisol levels among urban pregnant women. *Journal of Epidemiology and Community Health, 69*, 1169–1174. https://doi.org/10.1136/jech-2015-205541

Seng, J. S., Low, L. M. K., Sperlich, M., Ronis, D. L., & Liberzon, I. (2009). Prevalence, trauma history, and risk for posttraumatic stress disorder among nulliparous women in maternity care. *Obstetrics and Gynecology, 114*, 839. https://doi.org/10.1097/AOG.0b013e3181b8f8a2

Seth, S., Lewis, A. J., & Galbally, M. (2016). Perinatal maternal depression and cortisol function in pregnancy and the postpartum period: A systematic literature review. *BMC Pregnancy and Childbirth, 16*, 124. https://doi.org/10.1186/s12884-016-0915-y

Shadigian, E., & Bauer, S. T. (2005). Pregnancy-associated death: A qualitative systematic review of homicide and suicide. *Obstetrical & Gynecological Survey, 60*, 183–190. https://doi.org/10.1097/01.ogx.0000155967.72418.6b

Sheridan, M. A., & McLaughlin, K. A. (2014). Dimensions of early experience and neural development: Deprivation and threat. *Trends in Cognitive Sciences*, *18*, 580–585. https://doi.org/10.1016/j.tics.2014.09.001

Slade, A., & Cohen, L. J. (1996). The process of parenting and the remembrance of things past. *Infant Mental Health Journal*, *17*, 217–238. https://doi.org/10.1002/(SICI)1097-0355(199623)17:3<217::AID-IMHJ3>3.0.CO;2-L

Slade, A., Cohen, L. J., Sadler, L. S., & Miller, M. (2009). The psychology and psychopathology of pregnancy: Reorganization and transformation. In C. H. Zeanah (Ed.), *Handbook of infant mental health* (3rd ed., pp. 22–39). Guilford Press.

Sperlich, M., & Seng, J. S. (2008). *Survivor moms: Women's stories of birthing, mothering and healing after sexual abuse*. Motherbaby Press.

Sroufe, L. A. (2020). *A compelling idea: How we become the persons we are*. Safer Society Press.

Thompson, R. A. (2019). Emotion dysregulation: A theme in search of definition. *Development and Psychopathology*, *31*, 805–815. https://doi.org/10.1017/S0954579419000282

Tobin, V., & Delaney, K. R. (2019). Child abuse victimization among transgender and gender nonconforming people: A systematic review. *Perspectives in Psychiatric Care*, *55*, 576–583. https://doi.org/10.1111/ppc.12398

Yates, T. M., Carlson, E. A., & Egeland, B. (2008). A prospective study of child maltreatment and self-injurious behavior in a community sample. *Development and Psychopathology*, *20*, 651–671. https://doi.org/10.1017/S0954579408000321

Zhu, W., Chen, Y., & Xia, L. X. (2020). Childhood maltreatment and aggression: The mediating roles of hostile attribution bias and anger rumination. *Personality and Individual Differences*, *162*, 110007. https://doi.org/10.1016/j.paid.2020.110007

6

Child Abuse and Perinatal Outcomes: Examining Prenatal Health, Intergenerational Abuse, Motherhood, and Childbirth for Survivors

Eva Mohler and Robyn Brunton [ID]

Abstract This chapter provides an overview of outcomes related to child abuse that may be challenging for child abuse survivors during the perinatal period. In Part 1, general and psychological prenatal health is examined. This includes a discussion on prenatal substance use and eating disorders which have implications for the mother and child. Part 2 of this chapter examines motherhood, particularly the mother-child relationship and the intergenerational implications of child abuse. We discuss attachment, from its early prenatal development to postpartum bonding, and its importance for the infant in forming internal models of caregiving that, if impaired, can contribute to later mental health problems. The important role of breastfeeding in maternal bonding and the difficulties some survivors may encounter are also considered. Next, we examine the

E. Mohler
Saarland University Hospital, Homburg, Germany

R. Brunton (✉)
School of Psychology, Charles Sturt University, Bathurst, NSW, Australia
e-mail: rbrunton@csu.edu.au

© The Author(s), under exclusive license to Springer Nature Switzerland AG 2023
R. Brunton, R. Dryer (eds.), *Perinatal Care and Considerations for Survivors of Child Abuse*, https://doi.org/10.1007/978-3-031-33639-3_6

101

influence of previous child abuse on parenting practices and consider intergenerational abuse, that is, the potential of a mother with their own history of abuse to harm their child. Drawing on social learning theory and the parenting literature, it is clear that a parent's childhood experiences, which may include abuse and harsh parenting, are influential in their parenting practices. This part of the chapter concludes by considering child abuse survivors' risk of revictimization and the implications this risk poses for pregnant women and their unborn children. Indeed, pregnancy may increase the risk of IPV, and this violence can impact the mother and developing fetus through direct harm and epigenetic effects. The final part of this chapter examines the challenges of childbirth for survivors of childhood abuse and the importance of sensitive care. While childbirth can be particularly traumatizing for some survivors, empirical data suggest that positive birth experiences provide opportunities for caregivers to attenuate negative effects.

Keywords Prenatal eating disorder • Prenatal substance use • Attachment • Mother-child bonding • Revictimization • Intergenerational abuse • Childbirth

Child abuse is a global issue and, for some children, has long-term deleterious consequences (see Chap. 2 for definitions and prevalence) (Irish et al., 2010). Given the high incidence of child abuse in many countries, it is likely that a large proportion of women who become pregnant and have children will have a history of childhood abuse. This chapter provides an overview of certain outcomes related to child abuse that can present challenges for survivors during the perinatal period. In the first part of this chapter, we consider prenatal health, examining general and psychological health. This includes a discussion on prenatal substance use and eating disorders (ED) and the associated implications for mother and child. The second part examines the mother-child relationship from its early prenatal development to postpartum bonding and attachment. We also consider the influence of previous child abuse on parenting practices and intergenerational impacts. This part concludes by considering child abuse survivors' risk of being revictimized and the implications for pregnant women and their unborn children. The final part examines the childbirth experience for survivors of childhood abuse, including toko-phobia (i.e., fear of childbirth), and the importance of sensitive care. While we have not covered psychopathology in detail in this chapter, other chapters in this book specifically address anxiety, depression, suicide ideation, and PTSD (i.e., Chaps. 4 and 5).

Part 1. Prenatal Health

It is well established that the in-utero environment can have long-term implications for the unborn baby. Consistent with the fetal programming hypothesis or developmental origins of health and disease (Ellison, 2010), nutrition and environmental factors can alter development pathways during critical periods of prenatal development. In this first part on prenatal health, we consider the potential impact of child abuse on the mother and developing fetus.

General Health

During pregnancy, survivors of child abuse may experience poorer general health than other women. For example, in a case-control study of mother-infant pairs (matched for age and psychosocial status), women with a history of physical or sexual abuse had more pregnancy complications (e.g., severe vomiting), and their infants had more medical complications (e.g., feeding disorders) than other mothers (Möhler et al., 2008). Studies examining childhood sexual abuse, in particular, have identified that survivors may have more chronic pain, long-term health conditions (e.g., cardiopulmonary or gastrointestinal symptoms), and a greater likelihood of gynecological problems (e.g., genital tract infections) than other women (Brunton & Dryer, 2021; Irish et al., 2010). In addition, many survivors perceive their previous childhood abuse to negatively influence their prenatal care experience (Brunton & Dryer, 2021).

Concerningly, these health-related outcomes have consequences for the fetus. Specific conditions such as hypertension and diabetes increase the risk of preterm birth, low birth weight, placental abruption, congenital malformation, stillbirth, and miscarriage. Moreover, these health-related issues can contribute to perinatal complications and other procedures, such as a cesarean birth (Ali & Dornhorst, 2011, provide a review). These additional health issues likely increase prenatal care utilization and place additional demands on health systems.

Prenatal Substance Use

For some pregnant women, substance use contributes to these health-related issues. Substances such as alcohol, tobacco, and illicit drugs introduce harmful teratogens into the fetal environment and, even at low levels, can impact the growth and development of the fetus and contribute to adverse outcomes such as spontaneous abortion, preterm birth, and low birth weight (AIHW, 2020; Andersen et al., 2012). Moreover, being under the influence of alcohol or drugs while pregnant increases the risk of physical injury or harm due to impaired functioning (AIHW, 2020). The implications of longer-term substance use for the child include congenital disabilities, malformation (e.g., craniofacial abnormalities), developmental disorders, lower IQ, and, in some cases, a longer-term adverse sequela from fetal alcohol spectrum disorder (Keegan et al., 2010; Lewis et al., 2012). While most women decrease or eliminate alcohol when pregnant, a small percentage continue to consume alcohol despite the known risks (Brunton & Dryer, 2023; Meschke et al., 2003).

It is worth noting that research conducted in this area has been limited, with few studies examining child abuse specifically, and we therefore draw on the findings reported from research on adverse childhood experiences (ACEs). Despite this limitation, the findings predominantly confirm a relationship between childhood abuse and prenatal substance use. Racine et al. (2020) found that a history of family violence (i.e., physical abuse, emotional abuse, and domestic violence) nearly doubled the risk of prenatal binge drinking or smoking and increased the risk of drug taking by 1.5 times. A history of child sexual abuse increased the risk of drug use by 2.25 times. Frankenberger et al. (2015) noted a dose-response relationship between ACEs and pregnancy drinking. After adjusting for pre-pregnancy drinking and other demographics, experiencing one ACE increased the odds of drinking nearly threefold (aOR = 2.92), whereas four or more ACEs exponentially increased the risk to 4.8 times. Meschke et al. (2008) found that women who reported previous sexual abuse had 38% increased odds of prenatal drinking. However, while Osofsky et al. (2021) identified an increased risk for prenatal smoking, cannabis, and opioid use for those with ACEs (compared to no ACEs), the results for alcohol consumption were not statistically significant. Similarly, Brunton and Dryer's (2023) examination of 548 pregnant women found no relationship between childhood abuse and antenatal alcohol consumption. These inconsistencies may reflect methodological limitations such as samples with a low child abuse prevalence lacking the power to detect an effect (i.e., Brunton & Dryer, 2021), recruitment during antenatal care confounding accurate reporting of alcohol intake or by subsuming abuse and neglect under ACEs (i.e., Osofsky et al., 2021), which can mask individual findings. Notwithstanding this, evidence points to childhood abuse as a risk factor for prenatal substance use, with the severity of abuse potentially having a significant and negative influence on this relationship.

Psychological Health

In addition to physical health, a history of child abuse and, more broadly, early life maltreatment (ELM) is associated with a greater risk of psychopathology in the general population (Norman et al., 2012). Therefore, it is conceivable that pregnant women with a history of ELM will also be more susceptible to these psychological outcomes. Some of these particular outcomes are covered in more detail in Chap. 4 (PTSD) and Chap. 5 (depression, anxiety, and suicidality). In this chapter, we consider other psychological aspects with potentially high relevance for the perinatal period, that is, prenatal eating disorders.

Prenatal Eating Disorders (ED)

For victims of child abuse, there is reportedly an increased prevalence of ED (Rayworth et al., 2004). A global review estimated that the prevalence of ED for women in the general population is 3.3–18.6% (Galmiche et al., 2019). During pregnancy, maternal concern for the developing fetus can reduce ED symptoms (Crow et al., 2008); however, pregnant women with a child abuse history may be at greater risk of continued symptomology. One case-control study identified that women who met the criteria for an ED (i.e., bulimia, anorexia, or binge-eating) or reported ED symptoms were twice as likely to have a child physical abuse history. They were also over three times more likely to have a history of physical and sexual abuse in childhood (Rayworth et al., 2004). Among these women, severe abuse was associated with a threefold increase in ED diagnosis. These findings are consistent with previous research using larger samples (Senior et al., 2005). ED in pregnancy has also been associated with postnatal depression (Riesco-Gonzalez et al., 2022), thus potentially exacerbating the psychological issues of perinatal women with a history of child abuse.

ED can lead to malnutrition, electrolyte imbalances, anemia, and vitamin deficiencies for the mother (Sidiropoulos, 2007). These associated outcomes are of particular concern as an inadequate or restricted diet can harm the fetus. EDs in pregnancy are linked to poor fetal outcomes, including miscarriage, preterm birth, disabilities, and malformations (Sebastiani et al., 2020). In addition, fetal programming studies have identified that altered nutritional patterns, common among women with ED, can alter or influence epigenetic patterns (i.e., the expression of genes). These changes can trigger biological and psychological alterations in the offspring (e.g., a predisposition to chronic disease) that have long-term implications. Evidence on fetal programming and its implications for pregnant women is limited and requires further investigation. However, studies on pregnant women exposed to extreme hunger through war have shown an elevated risk of psychiatric disorders in their offspring (Ellison, 2010). Therefore, it is probable that the consequences of prenatal ED are long-term and intergenerational.

Part 2 Mother-Child Relationship

Mother-Child Bonding

In 1981, Cranley identified maternal-fetal attachment as the relationship that develops between a mother and her unborn baby. This relationship, seen as part of the normative developmental processes of pregnancy and motherhood (Alhusen, 2008), showed that the bond between the mother and child begins far earlier than attachment theorists such as Bowlby (1979) proposed. Since then, studies have examined the risk and protection of prenatal attachment, identifying factors such as mood disorders and family support, respectively (see Alhusen, 2008 for a critical review). However, studies examining whether childhood abuse influences this attachment relationship are limited.

Stark Stigger et al. (2020) found that childhood abuse or neglect negatively impacted maternal-fetal attachment. Emotional neglect and emotional abuse had the greatest impact on the attachment relationship, suggesting that these previous adverse emotional experiences may exert a more substantial impact on attachment through internalized negative self-beliefs (Wright et al., 2009). If the mother's childhood experience includes criticizing and rejecting experiences or an absence of socioemotional development (Glaser, 2002), this will likely influence their internalized beliefs and self-representations (Malone et al., 2010). These beliefs may disrupt normative development processes, including developing maternal self-representations (Malone et al., 2010). Given that maternal-fetal attachment is an important developmental task of pregnancy, it is conceivable that it would predict postnatal behavior and bonding; however, few studies have examined this (Alhusen, 2008).

Notwithstanding this, there is a plethora of research on mother-infant bonding (i.e., the affective tie between mother and child). The significance of this mother-child relationship was the focus of Bowlby and Ainsworth's early work on attachment (Bowlby, 1979). According to attachment theory, caregivers play a key role in the development of internal models of the relational world, and when impaired, parent-child bonding can be an influential factor in the pathogenesis of mental health problems (Otowa et al., 2013).

So far, findings support the association between poor parental bonding for abuse survivors and their offspring (Farre-Sender et al., 2018). Muzik et al. (2013) examined bonding six months postpartum in a sample of women with child abuse and neglect histories (N = 97) and women (N = 53) with no such history. While bonding disturbance was associated with prior child maltreatment, their findings indicated that psychopathology associated with maltreatment posed a greater risk to bonding than maltreatment alone. Moreover, and importantly, bonding impairment improved over time for all women regardless of their history, suggesting that bonding is a normative process independent of emotional disturbances.

In the early stages of the mother-child relationship, breastfeeding is an important aspect of maternal bonding. Breastfeeding has long-term health benefits for the mother and child (Victora et al., 2016) and contributes to early bonding and attachment (Linde et al., 2020). Regardless of child abuse history, women tend to have equal intentions to breastfeed (Elfgen et al., 2017); however, for many child abuse survivors, the intimacy of this experience, such as suckling or skin-to-skin contact, can trigger PTSD symptoms (e.g., disassociation or recurrence of traumatic memories) and influence their ability to persevere. Therefore, while many survivors may initiate breastfeeding, they may be unable to continue for extended periods (Coles et al., 2016; Elfgen et al., 2017).

Beyond the early bonding experience, child abuse survivors often report more parenting difficulties than others. Empirical evidence confirms more intrusive, impulsive, and hostile behaviors for women with physical or sexual abuse histories than other women (DiLillo & Damashek, 2003; Moehler et al., 2007). More broadly, studies into child abuse, neglect, and witnessing family violence confirm a link between ELM and maternal hostility toward their children (Bailey et al., 2012). Savage et al.'s (2019) meta-analysis (32 studies, 17,932 participants) demonstrated the negative impact of past abusive experiences on parenting behavior. Negative and potentially abusive parenting and parenting characterized by poor attachment/bonding had stronger relationships with ELM than positive parenting. More specifically, the relationship between emotional and/or physical abuse and parenting behavior was more robust than other abuse types (child sexual abuse was not statistically significant). The implications of impaired parenting behavior extend to the child's development and well-being such that these children may be more likely to have behavioral problems, poorer adult educational attainment, less positive social behavior, and greater negative affect and defiant noncompliance (Leerkes et al., 2009; Raby et al., 2015).

These intergenerational effects were demonstrated in a large-scale parenting study (N = 8292), which noted that mothers with a child sexual abuse history reported greater negativity and less maternal confidence in their relationship with their children (Roberts et al., 2004). Furthermore, compared to children of mothers with no abuse, the children of abused women had higher levels of hyperactivity and greater conduct, peer, and emotional problems. Additional analysis identified maternal anxiety and confidence mediated the relationship between the mother's sexual abuse history and children's conduct problems. These findings demonstrate the far-reaching consequences of child sexual abuse that extend into adulthood (mental health and parenting) and intergenerationally, showing that the relationship between prior abuse and parenting is complex.

Emotional availability is a key aspect of parenting behavior and may be altered by ELM. For example, research points to mothers who have experienced severe childhood abuse or those with remitted depression and a history of abuse being emotionally unavailable (i.e., less sensitivity, responsiveness, involvement) to their children compared to non-maltreated women (Fuchs et al., 2015; Moehler et al., 2007). Relatedly, the fast and accurate recognition and response to a child's emotional cues, such as facial expressions of emotions, may be altered for mothers with an ELM history. ELM-related alterations in the neural correlates of facial emotion processing were confirmed in a recent meta-analysis (20 studies, Hein & Monk, 2017) that found enhanced amygdala activation (a region associated with emotion) for maltreated individuals relative to controls. These findings suggest that ELM-related alterations may impact emotion regulation and increase the risk of later psychopathologies (i.e., depression, anxiety). Furthermore, ELM was associated with enhanced activations in other brain areas, such as the superior temporal gyrus (relative to controls), a region associated with social perception and cognition.

Therefore, while these ELM-related brain changes may be adaptive in childhood (by providing a means of identifying threatening emotions in their environment), they may impact their socioemotional functioning and, by extension, their parenting in later life.

Intergenerational Abuse

It has long been proposed that early experiences of child abuse can lead to the intergenerational transmission of abuse (Widom, 1989). That is, a mother abused in childhood may have greater potential to harm her child. One mechanism proposed for the intergenerational transmission of abuse is the mother's projection of negative self-representations onto their child (Möhler et al., 2001). This abuse transmission was illustrated in a case study describing a young mother with intense fears of her potential for violence. Her own abusive experiences, when projected onto her child, placed the child at greater risk of abuse, with the child's behavior interpreted as abusive toward the mother.

However, the literature specifically examining this intergenerational transmission of abuse is limited. Further, published studies are inconsistent in their findings. For instance, Appleyard et al. (2011) found that childhood physical or sexual abuse indirectly increased the risk of the mother abusing her child mediated by substance use. In contrast, Bert et al. (2009) noted that a history of childhood emotional abuse increased the potential for child abuse and a greater acceptance of abuse/neglect in first-time mothers. Childhood physical abuse similarly increased the risk for older mothers. Choi (2018) found that childhood emotional abuse indirectly influenced child harm exposure through postpartum depression but had no significant findings for childhood physical or sexual abuse. These differential outcomes may reflect a lack of sensitivity in the analyses (i.e., type II error), with some samples having a low prevalence of abuse types.

Despite these limited findings, that a parent's upbringing is influential in their parenting beliefs and behaviors is less disputed. Indeed, parents with a history of physical abuse are more likely to use punitive or harsh punishment, considered abusive (e.g., punching when angry), than those with mild physical abuse (Kim et al., 2010; Pears & Capaldi, 2001). Previous research also supports the hypothesis that a parent's level of functioning in their parent-child relationships is predicted by their experience of harsh parenting during their childhood (Brook et al., 2002; Conger et al., 2003). Theoretically, this is consistent with social learning theory, as victims of familial abuse would lack a positive parenting role model and thus have less opportunity to observe and model positive parenting (DiLillo & Damashek, 2003).

Revictimization

Consistent with the cycle of violence, a large body of evidence supports the proposition that childhood abuse is a risk factor for revictimization in the general population (Walker et al., 2019). This victimization, usually by an intimate partner, can be physical, sexual, emotional, or coercive control (WHO, 2011). For example, Butler et al. (2020) found that those who experienced childhood physical abuse were twice as likely (than controls) to experience past year violence and three times more likely to have experienced intimate partner violence (IPV) or sexual violence since 16 years of age. Furthermore, this risk increased exponentially relative to the frequency of childhood abuse (e.g., OR = 6.89 for multiple types of child abuse and sexual violence victimization). Moreover, in a recent meta-analysis of child maltreatment and IPV victimization (Li et al., 2019), differential effects were noted dependent on the child abuse type. These findings are consistent with theoretical explanations that propose that early sexual experiences increase a woman's vulnerability to later victimization through mechanisms such as traumatic sexualization (discussed in more detail in Chap. 3) or a propensity for higher alcohol use (Koss & Dinero, 1989).

Being pregnant is not a protection against IPV and may actually increase the risk for IPV in some instances. For example, pregnancy can create additional demands and stress on a relationship (e.g., increased financial concerns). Unwanted or unplanned pregnancies can further exacerbate this stress (Li et al., 2019; WHO, 2011). IPV experienced during pregnancy is of particular concern as it places both the mother and developing child at risk. Physical abuse is often targeted toward the woman's abdomen, potentially jeopardizing the pregnancy (WHO, 2011), and the physiological effects of stress associated with IPV can have epigenetic effects. These factors can contribute to preterm birth and increase the risk of miscarriage, perinatal death, and maternal mortality (WHO, 2013). Experiencing IPV during pregnancy has also been associated with increased negative health behaviors such as consuming alcohol, drugs, and smoking (WHO, 2011).

Childhood sexual abuse has been associated with a higher likelihood of lifetime and current IPV and is a risk factor for abuse in the current pregnancy. Pregnant women have been identified as having more than a two-fold increased risk of lifetime IPV (relative to no abuse), and multiple childhood abuse experiences increased this risk exponentially with more than a sevenfold risk of lifetime physical and sexual IPV (Barrios et al., 2015). Concerningly, the risk of experiencing IPV in the past year, which would include the current pregnancy, was more than threefold. Gartland et al. (2016), in an Australian study of 1507 nulliparous women, found that those who experienced physical or sexual abuse in childhood had increased odds of fearing their intimate partner during the current pregnancy (OR = 2.7 and 2.0, respectively). When assessed postpartum in the first year, these women with a child physical or sexual abuse history still had double the risk of experiencing any IPV.

There is also evidence to suggest that different childhood abuses are related to different types of IPV types during pregnancy. For example, Barnett et al. (2018) examined 832 pregnant women and found that childhood emotional abuse was a more potent risk factor for emotional IPV, and childhood physical and sexual abuse were stronger risk factors for physical IPV or sexual IPV (than emotional abuse and neglect). Barrios et al. (2015) noted that a history of child physical and sexual abuse increased the likelihood of experiencing physical and sexual IPV in the past year (aOR = 3.33). These findings suggest the importance of understanding the distinct effect of different abuses, as this knowledge may lead to more effective interventions in adulthood (Li et al., 2019).

Part 3. The Childbirth Experience

Studies into childhood sexual abuse have dominated research on child abuse and childbirth. Childbirth can trigger past abuse memories, which, for some, is the first reemergence of traumatic memories since childhood (Leeners et al., 2013). Post-traumatic stress reactions can occur when women with child sexual abuse experiences feel overwhelmed by the multiple procedures and intrusive vaginal exams that can occur during pregnancy (Leeners et al., 2016; Rhodes & Hutchinson, 1994). These experiences can be re-traumatizing, which can be understood as a recurring cycle for a pregnant woman with a history of sexual abuse. The cyclical nature of re-traumatization was conceptualized by Dallam (2010), who proposed four interrelated processes: threats of safety, exposure to triggers, post-traumatic stress reactions, and avoidant coping. For example, a woman sexually abused in childhood may become hypersensitive to threats of safety during situations where she feels vulnerable (e.g., during intrusive vaginal examinations) or lacks control, such as being in a position of powerlessness (Coles & Jones, 2009; Leeners et al., 2007). When triggered, women may dissociate to defend against feeling threatened and overwhelmed, with some women describing disassociation as helpful in suppressing unpleasant memories or emotions (Leeners et al., 2013). However, some women may avoid prenatal care visits as they fear re-traumatization or feel disillusioned or discouraged by previous encounters. Avoidant coping, however, is not optimal for their prenatal care.

Given these issues, it is unsurprising that many child abuse survivors fear childbirth. Women with a history of child abuse tend to have a stronger fear of childbirth (FoC) than other women. For example, Heimstad et al. (2006) found that pregnant women ($N = 1452$) who reported childhood physical or sexual abuse had greater FoC than non-abused women. However, no differences were observed for adult abuse. Lukasse et al. (2011) examined a large cohort of multiparous women ($N = 4876$) and found that child abuse was a risk factor for FoC in their second pregnancy, with the strongest risk being severe emotional abuse (aOR = 1.58). These prospective studies have modest effects, yet studies examining FoC by parity (i.e., multiparous and primiparous) show that a previous positive birth experience can potentially lessen FoC. Lukasse et al. (2010) found that for all child abuse types, the risk for severe FoC was stronger for primipara women than multipara women. That is, any child abuse (i.e., physical, sexual, or emotional) increased the odds of severe FoC for primiparas (OR = 2.48) and multiparas (OR = 1.50).

Moreover, the severity of abuse increased the odds exponentially for primiparous women (those who experienced multiple abuse experiences had a fivefold increased risk of severe FoC). However, the same dose-response result was not observed in multiparous women. Of interest, after adjusting for previous negative birth experiences for multiparous women, the risk for severe FoC was attenuated to nonsignificance, indicating that for these women, their FoC was related to a previous negative birth experience rather than to a history of child abuse.

This finding suggests that if primipara women have a positive birth experience, this may attenuate the impact of child abuse history on FoC in subsequent pregnancies. Therefore, given these associations between child abuse and childbirth and the opportunity that a positive birth experience may afford child abuse survivors, sensitive care is critical (see Chap. 7 for a comprehensive coverage of this issue). Health providers who may be emotionally unavailable or perceived as hostile or judgmental can exacerbate a woman's responses to care (Coles & Jones, 2009; Dallam, 2010). The implications of not providing sensitive care for child abuse survivors place them at increased risk of re-traumatization and avoidance of medical care (Coles & Jones, 2009; Dallam, 2010; Leeners et al., 2013).

Summary and Conclusion

Survivors of child abuse have a greater risk of poor prenatal health than other women. This includes general health with an increased risk for the propensity for prenatal substance use, potentially further exacerbating health-related issues. In addition, psychologically, survivors may be at a higher risk for continued ED symptomology, which can have far-reaching consequences for the unborn child. These risks may result in further prenatal care utilization. While the evidence does not point to a specific type of child abuse that predominantly increases these health risks, studies have generally focused on childhood sexual abuse for historical reasons (Chap. 2 reviews these reasons). However, the absence of evidence for physical and emotional abuse highlights the need for additional research. It is important to acknowledge that pregnancy could be a consequence of sexual abuse, and in such situations, there are severe implications for both the mother and unborn child (e.g., a higher likelihood of low maternal-fetal attachment and high levels of maternal distress). However, examining this issue was beyond the scope of this chapter.

Emotional abuse may be the most potent risk factor for poor relationship development or attachment due to the mother internalizing negative self-beliefs and representations. However, as shown by Muzik et al. (2013), bonding impairment is not fixed and can be improved over time, suggesting that the opportunity for positive interventions exists. Related to mother-child bonding is breastfeeding, and there is no difference between childhood abuse survivors and other women in their intention to breastfeed. However, despite these intentions, the physical experience can often be re-traumatizing, and survivors may not persevere.

In this chapter, we also examined the effect of child abuse on parenting practices. Given the findings presented, theoretical positions such as Bandura's social learning theory provide a basis for explaining these intergenerational impacts. Concerningly, child abuse is linked to more hostile parenting, and the consequences of this parenting (which in itself can be abusive) can result in conduct problems for the offspring of those parents. The intergenerational impact of child abuse is further indicated in studies examining abuse potential. Although limited evidence is available, previous child abuse is a risk factor for that child abusing their offspring in adulthood. Of course, these relationships are complex, and possible mediators include depression, substance use, and age. Again a mother's negative self-representations, internalized from the previous abuse, may also be a mechanism for this abuse potential.

Childhood abuse is also a risk factor for adulthood revictimization, and the implications of this can be far-reaching when experienced during pregnancy. In some cases, the risks may be exacerbated by additional stressors of pregnancy. In addition, research evidence suggests a differential risk with certain abuse types, increasing the risk for certain IPV types in adulthood. These findings highlight the importance of examining different types of child abuse and their differential effect, as it can assist in developing more effective interventions.

Childbirth can be challenging for child abuse survivors, and some survivors have a severe fear of it. Again this has been studied predominantly for survivors of child sexual abuse. However, Dallam's model, which was developed specifically for child sexual abuse, helps understand the concerns of all abuse survivors. For example, concerns around safety, triggers, post-traumatic reactions, and using avoidance-coping are likely common to all child abuse survivors. In addition, FoC can be common among primipara women with previous abuse histories. However, a positive birth experience provides an opportunity to intervene for subsequent pregnancies.

Based on the evidence presented in this chapter, the need for sensitive care is evident. Sensitive care affords many opportunities to intervene between the ongoing impact of child abuse and these perinatal outcomes. Pregnancy and childbirth are vulnerable periods in the life of women with past child abuse experiences. Addressing this concern and creating a trauma-sensitive pre- and peripartum environment can prevent maternal retraumatization and contribute to a healthier parent-child interaction.

References

AIHW. (2020). *Alcohol, tobacco & other drugs in Australia.* https://www.aihw.gov.au/reports/alcohol/alcohol-tobacco-other-drugs-australia

Alhusen, J. L. (2008). A literature update on maternal-fetal attachment. *Journal of Obstetric, Gynecologic & Neonatal Nursing, 37*(3), 315–328. https://doi.org/10.1111/j.1552-6909.2008.00241.x

Ali, S., & Dornhorst, A. (2011). Diabetes in pregnancy: Health risks and management. *Postgraduate Medical Journal, 87*(1028), 417–427. https://doi.org/10.1136/pgmj.2010.109157

Andersen, A.-M. N., Andersen, P. K., Olsen, J., Grønbæk, M., & Strandberg-Larsen, K. (2012). Moderate alcohol intake during pregnancy and risk of fetal death. *International Journal of Epidemiology, 41*(2), 405–413. https://doi.org/10.1093/ije/dyr189

Appleyard, K., Berlin, L., Rosanbalm, K., & Dodge, K. (2011). Preventing early child maltreatment: Implications from a longitudinal study of maternal abuse history, substance use problems, and offspring victimization. *Prevention Science, 12*(2), 139–149. https://doi.org/10.1007/s11121-010-0193-2

Bailey, H. N., DeOliveira, C. A., Wolfe, V. V., Evans, E. M., & Hartwick, C. (2012). The impact of childhood maltreatment history on parenting: A comparison of maltreatment types and assessment methods. *Child Abuse & Neglect, 36*(3), 236–246. https://doi.org/10.1016/j.chiabu.2011.11.005

Barnett, W., Halligan, S., Heron, J., Fraser, A., Koen, N., Zar, H. J., Donald, K. A., & Stein, D. J. (2018). Maltreatment in childhood and intimate partner violence: A latent class growth analysis in a South African pregnancy cohort. *Child Abuse & Neglect, 86*, 336–348. https://doi.org/10.1016/j.chiabu.2018.08.020

Barrios, Y. V., Gelaye, B., Zhong, Q., Nicolaidis, C., Rondon, M. B., Garcia, P. J., Sanchez, P. A., Sanchez, S. E., & Williams, M. A. (2015). Association of childhood physical and sexual abuse with intimate partner violence, poor general health and depressive symptoms among pregnant women. *PLoS One, 10*(1), e0116609. https://doi.org/10.1371/journal.pone.0116609

Bert, S. C., Guner, B. M., Lanzi, R. G., & Neglect, C. P. C. (2009). The influence of maternal history of abuse on parenting knowledge and behavior. *Family Relations, 58*(2), 176–187. https://doi.org/10.1111/j.1741-3729.2008.00545.x

Bowlby, J. (1979). The Bowlby-Ainsworth attachment theory. *Behavioral and Brain Sciences, 2*(4), 637–638.

Brook, J. S., Whiteman, M., & Zheng, L. (2002). Intergenerational transmission of risks for problem behavior. *Journal of Abnormal Child Psychology, 30*(1), 65–76. https://doi.org/10.1023/A:1014283116104

Brunton, R., & Dryer, R. (2021). Child sexual abuse and pregnancy: A systematic review of the literature. *Child Abuse & Neglect, 111*, 104802. https://doi.org/10.1016/j.chiabu.2020.104802

Brunton, R., & Dryer, R. (2023). Alcohol consumption after pregnancy awareness and the additive effect of pregnancy-related anxiety and child abuse. *Current Psychology*. https://doi.org/10.1007/s12144-023-04387-6

Butler, N., Quigg, Z., & Bellis, M. A. (2020). Cycles of violence in England and Wales: The contribution of childhood abuse to risk of violence revictimisation in adulthood. *BMC Medicine, 18*(1), 1–13. https://doi.org/10.1186/s12916-020-01788-3

Choi, K. W. (2018). *Postpartum depression in the intergenerational transmission of child maltreatment: Longitudinal evidence from global settings*. Dissertation Abstracts International: Section B: The Sciences and Engineering, 78(12-B).

Coles, J., Anderson, A., & Loxton, D. (2016). Breastfeeding duration after childhood sexual abuse: An Australian cohort study. *Journal of Human Lactation, 32*(3), NP28–NP35. https://doi.org/10.1177/0890334415590782

Coles, J., & Jones, K. (2009). "Universal precautions": Perinatal touch and examination after childhood sexual abuse. *Birth, 36*(3), 230–236. https://doi.org/10.1111/j.1523-536X.2009.00327.x

Conger, R. D., Neppl, T., Kim, K. J., & Scaramella, L. (2003). Angry and aggressive behavior across three generations: A prospective, longitudinal study of parents and children. *Journal of Abnormal Child Psychology, 31*(2), 143–160. https://doi.org/10.1023/a:1022570107457

Cranley, M. S. (1981). Development of a tool for the measurement of maternal attachment during pregnancy. *Nursing Research, 30*(5), 281–284.

Crow, S. J., Agras, W. S., Crosby, R., Halmi, K., & Mitchell, J. E. (2008). Eating disorder symptoms in pregnancy: A prospective study. *International Journal of Eating Disorders, 41*(3), 277–279. https://doi.org/10.1002/eat.20496

Dallam, S. J. (2010). A model of the retraumatization process: A meta-synthesis of childhood sexual abuse survivors' experiences in healthcare. *Dissertation Abstracts International: Section B: The Sciences and Engineering, 71*(2-B), 920.

DiLillo, D., & Damashek, A. (2003). Parenting characteristics of women reporting a history of childhood sexual abuse. *Child Maltreatment, 8*(4), 319–333. https://doi.org/10.1177/1077559503257104

Elfgen, C., Hagenbuch, N., Gorres, G., Block, E., & Leeners, B. (2017). Breastfeeding in women having experienced childhood sexual abuse. *Journal of Human Lactation, 33*(1), 119–127. https://doi.org/10.1177/0890334416680789

Ellison, P. T. (2010). Fetal programming and fetal psychology. *Infant and Child Development, 19*(1), 6–20. https://doi.org/10.1002/icd.649

Farre-Sender, B., Torres, A., Gelabert, E., Andres, S., Roca, A., Lasheras, G., Valdes, M., & Garcia-Esteve, L. (2018). Mother-infant bonding in the postpartum period: Assessment of the impact of pre-delivery factors in a clinical sample. *Archives of Women's Mental Health, 21*(3), 287–297. https://doi.org/10.1007/s00737-017-0785-y

Frankenberger, D. J., Clements-Nolle, K., & Yang, W. (2015). The association between adverse childhood experiences and alcohol use during pregnancy in a representative sample of adult women. *Women's Health Issues, 25*(6), 688–695. https://doi.org/10.1016/j.whi.2015.06.007

Fuchs, A., Mohler, E., Resch, F., & Kaess, M. (2015). Impact of a maternal history of childhood abuse on the development of mother-infant interaction during the first year of life. *Child Abuse & Neglect, 48,* 179–189. https://doi.org/10.1016/j.chiabu.2015.05.023

Galmiche, M., Déchelotte, P., Lambert, G., & Tavolacci, M. P. (2019). Prevalence of eating disorders over the 2000–2018 period: A systematic literature review. *The American Journal of Clinical Nutrition, 109*(5), 1402–1413. https://doi.org/10.1093/ajcn/nqy342

Gartland, D., Woolhouse, H., Giallo, R., McDonald, E., Hegarty, K., Mensah, F., Herrman, H., & Brown, S. J. (2016). Vulnerability to intimate partner violence and poor mental health in the first 4-year postpartum among mothers reporting childhood abuse: An Australian pregnancy cohort study. *Archives of Women's Mental Health, 19*(6), 1091–1100. https://doi.org/10.1007/s00737-016-0659-8

Glaser, D. (2002). Emotional abuse and neglect (psychological maltreatment): A conceptual framework. *Child Abuse & Neglect, 26*(6), 697–714. https://doi.org/10.1016/S0145-2134(02)00342-3

Heimstad, R., Dahloe, R., Laache, I., Skogvoll, E., & Schei, B. (2006). Fear of childbirth and history of abuse: Implications for pregnancy and delivery. *Acta Obstetricia et Gynecologica Scandinavica, 85*(4), 435–440. https://doi.org/10.1080/00016340500432507

Hein, T. C., & Monk, C. S. (2017). Research review: Neural response to threat in children, adolescents, and adults after child maltreatment - A quantitative meta-analysis. *Journal of Child Psychology and Psychiatry, 58*(3), 222–230. https://doi.org/10.1111/jcpp.12651

Irish, L., Kobayashi, I., & Delahanty, D. L. (2010). Long-term physical health consequences of childhood sexual abuse: A meta-analytic review. *Journal of Pediatric Psychology, 35*(5), 450–461. https://doi.org/10.1093/jpepsy/jsp118

Keegan, J., Parva, M., Finnegan, M., Gerson, A., & Belden, M. (2010). Addiction in pregnancy. *Journal of Addictive Diseases, 29*(2), 175–191. https://doi.org/10.1080/10550881003684723

Kim, H. K., Pears, K. C., Fisher, P. A., Connelly, C. D., & Landsverk, J. A. (2010). Trajectories of maternal harsh parenting in the first 3 years of life. *Child Abuse & Neglect, 34*(12), 897–906. https://doi.org/10.1016/j.chiabu.2010.06.002

Koss, M. P., & Dinero, T. E. (1989). Discriminant analysis of risk factors for sexual victimization among a national sample of college women. *Journal of Consulting and Clinical Psychology, 57*(2), 242. https://doi.org/10.1037/0022-006X.57.2.242

Leeners, B., Gorres, G., Block, E., & Hengartner, M. P. (2016). Birth experiences in adult women with a history of childhood sexual abuse. *Journal of*

Psychosomatic Research, 83, 27–32. https://doi.org/10.1016/j. jpsychores.2016.02.006

Leeners, B., Stiller, R., Block, E., Görres, G., Imthurn, B., & Rath, W. (2007). Effect of childhood sexual abuse on gynecologic care as an adult. *Psychosomatics, 48*(5), 385–393. https://doi.org/10.1176/appi.psy.48.5.385

Leeners, B., Stiller, R., Block, E., Gorres, G., Rath, W., & Tschudin, S. (2013). Prenatal care in adult women exposed to childhood sexual abuse. *Journal of Perinatal Medicine, 41*(4), 365–374. https://doi.org/10.1515/jpm-2011-0086

Leerkes, E. M., Blankson, A. N., & O'Brien, M. (2009). Differential effects of maternal sensitivity to infant distress and nondistress on social-emotional functioning. *Child Development, 80,* 762–775. https://doi.org/10.1111/j.1467-8624.2009.01296.x

Lewis, S. J., Zuccolo, L., Davey Smith, G., Macleod, J., Rodriguez, S., Draper, E. S., Barrow, M., Alati, R., Sayal, K., & Ring, S. (2012). Fetal alcohol exposure and IQ at age 8: Evidence from a population-based birth-cohort study. *PLoS One, 7*(11), e49407. https://doi.org/10.1371/journal.pone.0049407

Li, S., Zhao, F., & Yu, G. (2019). Childhood maltreatment and intimate partner violence victimization: A meta-analysis. *Child Abuse & Neglect, 88,* 212–224. https://doi.org/10.1016/j.chiabu.2018.11.012

Linde, K., Lehnig, F., Nagl, M., & Kersting, A. (2020). The association between breastfeeding and attachment: A systematic review. *Midwifery, 81,* 102592. https://doi.org/10.1016/j.midw.2019.102592

Lukasse, M., Vangen, S., Oian, P., Kumle, M., Ryding, E. L., & Schei, B. (2010). Childhood abuse and fear of childbirth-a population-based study. *Birth: Issues in Perinatal Care, 37*(4), 267–274. https://doi.org/10.1111/j.1523-536X.2010.00420.x

Lukasse, M., Vangen, S., Øian, P., & Schei, B. (2011). Fear of childbirth, women's preference for cesarean section and childhood abuse: A longitudinal study. *Acta Obstetricia et Gynecologica Scandinavica, 90*(1), 33–40. https://doi.org/10.1111/j.1600-0412.2010.01024.x

Malone, J. C., Levendosky, A. A., Dayton, C. J., & Bogat, G. A. (2010). Understanding the "ghosts in the nursery" of pregnant women experiencing domestic violence: Prenatal maternal representations and histories of childhood maltreatment. *Infant Mental Health Journal, 31*(4), 432–454. https://doi.org/10.1002/imhj.20264

Meschke, L. L., Hellerstedt, W., Holl, J. A., & Messelt, S. (2008). Correlates of prenatal alcohol use. *Maternal and Child Health Journal, 12*(4), 442–451. https://doi.org/10.1007/s10995-007-0261-9

Meschke, L. L., Holl, J. A., & Messelt, S. (2003). Assessing the risk of fetal alcohol syndrome: Understanding substance use among pregnant women. *Neurotoxicology and Teratology, 25*(6), 667–674. https://doi.org/10.1016/j. ntt.2003.07.004

Moehler, E., Biringen, Z., & Poustka, L. (2007). Emotional availability in a sample of mothers with a history of abuse. *American Journal of Orthopsychiatry, 77*(4), 624–628. https://doi.org/10.1037/0002-9432.77.4.624

Möhler, E., Matheis, V., Marysko, M., Finke, P., Kaufmann, C., Cierpka, M., Reck, C., & Resch, F. (2008). Complications during pregnancy, peri- and postnatal period in a sample of women with a history of child abuse. *Journal of Psychosomatic Obstetrics and Gynecology, 29*(3), 197–202. https://doi. org/10.1080/01674820801934252

Möhler, E., Resch, F., Cierpka, A., & Cierpka, M. (2001). The early appearance and intergenerational transmission of maternal traumatic experiences in the context of mother-infant interaction. *Journal of Child Psychotherapy, 27*(3), 257–271. https://doi.org/10.1080/00754170127346

Muzik, M., Bocknek, E. L., Broderick, A., Richardson, P., Rosenblum, K. L., Thelen, K., & Seng, J. S. (2013). Mother-infant bonding impairment across the first 6 months postpartum: The primacy of psychopathology in women with childhood abuse and neglect histories. *Archives of Women's Mental Health, 16*(1), 29–38. https://doi.org/10.1007/s00737-012-0312-0

Norman, R. E., Byambaa, M., De, R., Butchart, A., Scott, J., & Vos, T. (2012). The long-term health consequences of child physical abuse, emotional abuse, and neglect: A systematic review and meta-analysis. *PLoS Medicine, 9*(11), e1001349. https://doi.org/10.1371/journal.pmed.1001349

Osofsky, J. D., Osofsky, H. J., Frazer, A. L., Fields-Olivieri, M. A., Many, M., Selby, M., Holman, S., & Conrad, E. (2021). The importance of adverse childhood experiences during the perinatal period. *The American Psychologist, 76*(2), 350–363. https://doi.org/10.1037/amp0000770

Otowa, T., Gardner, C. O., Kendler, K. S., & Hettema, J. M. (2013). Parenting and risk for mood, anxiety and substance use disorders: A study in population-based male twins. *Social Psychiatry and Psychiatric Epidemiology, 48*(11), 1841–1849. https://doi.org/10.1007/s00127-013-0656-4

Pears, K. C., & Capaldi, D. M. (2001). Intergenerational transmission of abuse: A two-generational prospective study of an at-risk sample. *Child Abuse & Neglect, 25*, 1439–1461. https://doi.org/10.1016/S0145-2134(01)00286-1

Raby, K. L., Roisman, G. I., Fraley, R. C., & Simpson, J. A. (2015). The enduring predictive significance of early maternal sensitivity: Social and academic competence through age 32 years. *Child Development, 86*(3), 695–708. https://doi.org/10.1111/cdev.12325

Racine, N., McDonald, S., Chaput, K., Tough, S., & Madigan, S. (2020). Maternal substance use in pregnancy: Differential prediction by childhood adversity subtypes. *Preventative Medicine, 141,* 106303. https://doi.org/10.1016/j.ypmed.2020.106303

Rayworth, B. B., Wise, L. A., & Harlow, B. L. (2004). Childhood abuse and risk of eating disorders in women. *Epidemiology, 15*(3), 271–278. https://doi.org/10.1097/01.ede.0000120047.07140.9d

Rhodes, N., & Hutchinson, S. (1994). Labor experiences of childhood sexual abuse survivors. *Birth, 21*(4), 213–220. https://doi.org/10.1111/j.1523-536X.1994.tb00532.x

Riesco-Gonzalez, F. J., Antunez-Calvente, I., Vazquez-Lara, J. M., Rodriguez-Diaz, L., Palomo-Gomez, R., Gomez-Salgado, J., Garcia-Iglesias, J. J., Parron-Carreno, T., & Fernandez-Carrasco, F. J. (2022). Body image dissatisfaction as a risk factor for postpartum depression. *Medicina (Kaunas, Lithuania), 58*(6). https://doi.org/10.3390/medicina58060752

Roberts, R., O'Connor, T., Dunn, J., Golding, J., & Team, A. S. (2004). The effects of child sexual abuse in later family life; mental health, parenting and adjustment of offspring. *Child Abuse & Neglect, 28*(5), 525–545. https://doi.org/10.1016/j.chiabu.2003.07.006

Savage, L. E., Tarabulsy, G. M., Pearson, J., Collin-Vezina, D., & Gagne, L. M. (2019). Maternal history of childhood maltreatment and later parenting behavior: A meta-analysis. *Development and Psychopathology, 31*(1), 9–21. https://doi.org/10.1017/S0954579418001542

Sebastiani, G., Andreu-Fernandez, V., Herranz Barbero, A., Aldecoa-Bilbao, V., Miracle, X., Meler Barrabes, E., Balada Ibanez, A., Astals-Vizcaino, M., Ferrero-Martinez, S., Gomez-Roig, M. D., & Garcia-Algar, O. (2020). Eating disorders during gestation: Implications for Mother's health, fetal outcomes, and epigenetic changes. *Frontiers in Pediatrics, 8,* 587. https://doi.org/10.3389/fped.2020.00587

Senior, R., Barnes, J., Emberson, J. R., Golding, J., & Team, A. S. (2005). Early experiences and their relationship to maternal eating disorder symptoms, both lifetime and during pregnancy. *The British Journal of Psychiatry, 187,* 268–273. https://www.cambridge.org/core

Sidiropoulos, M. (2007). Anorexia nervosa: The physiological consequences of starvation and the need for primary prevention efforts. *McGill Journal of*

Medicine, *10*(1), 20–25. https://www.ncbi.nlm.nih.gov/pmc/articles/ PMC2323541/

Stark Stigger, R., de Souza Ribeiro Martinsa, C., Bonati de Matosa, M., Puchalski Trettima, J., Kurz da Cunhaa, G., Coelho Scholl, C., Pereira Ramosa, M., dos Santos Mottaa, J. V., Ghisleni, G., Tavares Pinheiro, R., & de Avila Quevedoa, L. (2020). Is maternal exposure to childhood trauma associated with maternal-fetal attachment? *Interpersona,* *14*(2), 200–210. https://doi.org/10.5964/ijpr.v14i2.3983

Victora, C. G., Bahl, R., Barros, A. J., França, G. V., Horton, S., Krasevec, J., Murch, S., Sankar, M. J., Walker, N., & Rollins, N. C. (2016). Breastfeeding in the 21st century: Epidemiology, mechanisms, and lifelong effect. *The Lancet,* *387*(10017), 475–490. https://www.thelancet.com/journals/lancet/ article/PIIS0140-6736(15)01024-7/fulltext.

Walker, H. E., Freud, J. S., Ellis, R. A., Fraine, S. M., & Wilson, L. C. (2019). The prevalence of sexual revictimization: A meta-analytic review. *Trauma, Violence, & Abuse,* *20*(1), 67–80. https://doi.org/10.1177/1524838017692364

WHO. (2011). *Intimate partner violence during pregnancy.* https://apps.who.int/ iris/bitstream/handle/10665/70764/WHO_RHR_11.35_eng.pdf

WHO. (2013). *Global and regional estimates of violence against women: Prevalence and health effects of intimate partner violence and non-partner sexual violence* (9241564628). https://www.who.int/publications/i/item/9789241564625

Widom, C. S. (1989). Does violence beget violence? A critical examination of the literature. *Psychological Bulletin,* *106*(1), 3–28. https://doi.org/ 10.1037/0033-2909.106.1.3

Wright, M. O. D., Crawford, E., & Del Castillo, D. (2009). Childhood emotional maltreatment and later psychological distress among college students: The mediating role of maladaptive schemas. *Child Abuse & Neglect,* *33*(1), 59–68. https://doi.org/10.1016/j.chiabu.2008.12.007

7

Screening for Child Abuse and Trauma During the Perinatal Period

Mickey Sperlich ⓘ and Whitney E. Mendel ⓘ

Abstract Given established links between child abuse and adverse perinatal effects, many professional organizations recommend screening. Screening provides opportunities to identify survivors who may benefit from interventions and tailor care that minimizes eliciting trauma triggers and prevents re-traumatization. However, there are both client- and provider-level barriers to screening. Conditions that foster disclosures include the application of provider trauma sensitivity and use of culturally congruent screening tools. Screening should be regarded as part of a continuum of trauma responsivity that includes training, preparation, screening, offering referrals and interventions, and evaluating care. Several tools are available to screen for child abuse and other trauma and

M. Sperlich (✉)
University at Buffalo, School of Social Work, Buffalo, NY, USA
e-mail: msperlic@buffalo.edu

W. E. Mendel
Roswell Park Comprehensive Cancer Center, Buffalo, NY, USA

their sequelae. Basic recommendations across screening contexts include careful preparation and education on the part of the provider, identifying optimal procedures for implementation, establishing good rapport, identifying any provider self-triggers and establishing workplace support including reflective supervision, developing normalizing preamble language prior to screening, connecting past trauma to the present, addressing confidentiality, being an active listener, validating, empathizing, and showing support, "right-sizing" provider response, and making appropriate referrals. Finally, perinatal screening for child abuse must proceed in tandem with the creation, evaluation, and availability of trauma-specific interventions. *Why* we screen is clear; *how* to screen bears elucidation.

Keywords Perinatal screening recommendations • Screening tools • Continuum of trauma responsivity • Cultural congruency • Trauma-informed perinatal care • Trauma disclosure • Prevention of retraumatization

In this chapter, we present the arguments for and against child abuse screening during the childhood period, the current screening landscape, the need for a continuum of trauma-informed responsivity, a brief review of existing tools, and basic recommendations and precautions. It is widely recognized that experiences of child abuse (e.g., sexual abuse, physical abuse, neglect) are adverse childhood experiences (ACEs) that often impose consequences to the physical and mental health across the life span of the survivor (Felitti et al., 1998). In the context of the perinatal period, ripple effects of child abuse may not only impact the birthing person in their experience of pregnancy, labor, delivery, and postpartum (Hutchens et al., 2017; Seng et al., 2009), they may extend beyond the individual, for example, by increasing risk for pregnancy complications (Leeners et al., 2010), as well as shorter length of gestation and lower birthweight of the infant born to the survivor (Seng et al., 2011). Further still, consequences of experiences of child abuse have been found to potentially impair bonding between the birthing parent and their infant (Muzik et al., 2013; Seng et al., 2013; Souch et al., 2022), and affect parenting styles more broadly (Newcomb & Locke, 2001), which may result in increased vulnerability of the child(ren) experiencing trauma of their own as part of intergenerational cycles of abuse. Given the prevalence of histories of child abuse in the population and the probable reach of consequences across generations, it is incumbent upon perinatal providers to consider the role of screening for histories of child abuse as part of care for pregnant and parenting individuals.

While screening for histories of child abuse among pregnant individuals is recommended by professional organizations, such as the American College of Obstetricians and Gynecologists (ACOG, 2011), to screen or not to screen remains an openly debated question. The potential benefits of prenatal screening have been enumerated. Perinatal providers are uniquely positioned to potentially interrupt the intergenerational transmission of ACEs, including child abuse. Screening has been suggested to aid in mitigating the ramifications of child abuse and connecting individuals to needed resources (Atzl et al., 2019). Others suggest that screening prenatally may help clinicians monitor for postpartum depression, creating an opportunity for more open dialogue in the postpartum period and, therefore, more timely support (Hutchens et al., 2017).

With the growing recognition of proximal and distal impacts that may result from child abuse, studies have also explored the acceptability of being screened among pregnant and newly parenting individuals. Flanagan et al. (2018) found that, among the participants in their pilot study, most accepted screening for ACEs, a common tool for assessing experiences of child abuse, and found that discussing ACEs with their provider improved perceptions of their relationship with their provider. Olsen et al. (2021) indicated that most birthing persons in their study supported prenatal screening for ACEs. Similarly, Watson et al. (2021) found that individuals in their sample valued conversations about ACEs and suggested that such conversations should be part of standard prenatal care. In fact, those with higher ACE scores in their sample were more likely to desire a lengthier conversation with their provider. Mersky et al. (2019) also reported that the vast majority of individuals who participated in a home visiting program were not at all uncomfortable, or only slightly uncomfortable, completing the ACE questionnaire. In some instances, individuals found comfort in being screened, such as in a small cross-sectional study conducted by Lee et al. (2012) in a general practice setting with female participants who had experienced child abuse. Findings from this study indicated that more than half of those who participated felt relieved and hopeful when their general practitioner asked about their experiences of child abuse.

In a pilot study conducted by Flanagan et al. (2018), prenatal screening for ACEs was found to increase comfort among providers in discussing ACEs, providing education about the consequences of ACEs, and referring to appropriate resources. In addition, Flanagan et al. (2018) found that implementing screening in a clinical setting was feasible and acceptable among clinicians when they were adequately trained and provided with appropriate referral resources. In a systematic review of the literature, Rariden et al. (2021) found that discussing ACEs with patients generated a better understanding of the patient and promoted empathy among providers. The benefits of screening have also been suggested to help identify potential triggers to past trauma and thereby help prevent retraumatization in the prenatal period (Millar et al., 2021; Sperlich et al., 2017).

It is important to note that support for screening in the aforementioned studies is not without its limitations. Our understanding of how best to support survivors of abuse in childhood trails behind our understanding of the sequelae resulting from childhood trauma and adversity. Research specific to screening for a history of child abuse is in its infancy and is only available at the speed of uptake of screening practices in perinatal care. Despite such limitations, as evidenced above, screening as part of perinatal care shows promise to the birthing person, their child(ren), and providers.

Challenges and Barriers Related to Screening

While there is mounting evidence regarding the benefits of prenatal screening for histories of child abuse, challenges remain for providers and clients alike. These include irregular screening practices by clinicians, clinician discomfort, fear of causing distress, and inadequate referral and support resources. Farrow et al. (2018) surveyed 145 obstetrician-gynecologists (OB-GYNs) regarding prenatal screening for histories of abuse.

While the vast majority of respondents acknowledged the importance of such screening, few indicated that they regularly screen their patients, and one-third of OB-GYNs indicated that they never screen for histories of abuse. Unpacking what prevents OB-GYNs from screening their patients, Farrow et al. (2018) found that some of the most noted barriers include insufficient time to screen and counsel patients, the lack of a system of care in place for those who need help, inadequate support staff, and contradictory recommendations for screening and intervention. Additional barriers to screening practices noted by Farrow et al. (2018) are born out of clinician discomfort, specifically not knowing how to screen or what to do if a person discloses abuse. These mirror findings regarding screening for past trauma and domestic violence in a large perinatal study (Seng et al., 2008) and are echoed in Maunder et al.'s (2020) work among a broad swath of clinicians, including primary care physicians, psychiatrists, and specialists. Clinicians surveyed in the Maunder et al. (2020) study also reported a lack of time to screen, concerns regarding a lack of mental health support in place, and a lack of confidence in screening as barriers. These findings are consistent with those noted among pediatricians and primary care providers in screening for postpartum depression among new parents at well-child visits and within the first year postpartum (Docherty et al., 2020; Yu & Sampson, 2019).

Another barrier noted among some perinatal providers is a fear of causing distress among patients by screening (Maunder et al., 2020). This concern extends beyond histories of trauma in childhood and is often indicated among providers when asking about other topics deemed sensitive, such as intimate partner violence (IPV) and psychosis (Carroll et al., 2018). An oath of doing no harm may constitute a barrier to screening for histories of child abuse or current circumstances of abuse among providers. There is evidence to suggest that screening for histories of child abuse may result in discomfort for some. While Mersky et al. (2019) noted that most individuals in their study (80%) experienced little to no discomfort completing the ACE questionnaire, they did find that 3% of their study sample, particularly those with higher ACE scores, reported considerable discomfort. Importantly, Mersky et al. (2019) also found a relationship between provider discomfort and client discomfort, such that any degree of provider discomfort with the ACE questionnaire was associated with a higher degree of discomfort for the client. Similarly, Gokhale et al. (2020) reported mixed findings regarding screening among the small sample of women they interviewed, with nearly half of their sample reporting that screening may be beneficial, while others reported fear of re-traumatization or they simply did not believe the relevance of past trauma in their current pregnancy. In a longitudinal study by Seng et al. (2008), pregnant survivors of abuse identified through the research study reported disclosing to their perinatal providers at much lower rates than they disclosed to the researchers; although the vast majority thought that their provider did a good job of asking, reasons for nondisclosures included the perception that disclosing to perinatal providers would not have been relevant or helpful, or would be too painful. Much like the subjectivity inherent in defining what is and what is not traumatic for individuals, there appears to be considerable subjectivity related to the perceived impact and relevance of screening.

These challenges to screening are situated in a larger context of ethical and logistical considerations of the practice of screening. To screen or not to screen is not the only question. If we are to screen, questions of when to screen, who should screen, and how to screen are among some of the most pressing. Thackeray et al. (2007) explored experiences of screening among women who had experienced IPV and found there is a preference to be screened by someone of the same gender, race, and relatively close in age. Mendel et al. (2021) raise concerns about the administration of a screening tool, noting a lack of trauma-informed practices in the screening process, which may lead to re-traumatization. Finkelhor (2018) poses yet another question, "What supports are needed if we are to screen?" Finkelhor (2018), a prominent voice illuminating the broad challenges to public health screening practices, cautions it is premature to implement universal screening of ACEs, imploring us to consider what must be in place before we screen. Ethically, he questions whether it is reasonable to screen when there is no guarantee of the availability of proper treatment, particularly for those with high ACE scores. He suggests that those with high ACE scores may have far more complex needs, complicating what treatment is most appropriate, prescribed, and available. McLennan et al. (2020) further this concern by questioning the consequences of labeling an individual "high-risk" and the lack of availability or access to effective treatment options once labeled as such. Finkelhor (2018) also asks us to consider potential negative consequences that may emerge from screening, such as the risk of overtreatment potentially resulting in an increased burden on behavioral health systems. He encourages us to question what makes the most sense (and is evidence-based): to be screening for ACEs themselves, or for possible health behaviors that may result from a history of ACEs, such as substance use and other maladaptive coping strategies.

While there is much yet to learn, challenges to screening, and mixed evidence regarding the acceptability and utility of screening for histories of child abuse among both perinatal providers and the individuals seeking care, there are numerous current efforts to screen for histories of child abuse in the perinatal period. Best practices are emerging from which we can draw insight and move forward in better supporting perinatal providers in screening practices and evolving necessary resources to better meet the needs of individuals in the perinatal period living with histories of child abuse.

Current Screening Landscape

Professional perinatal organizations recommend screening in various ways. In addition to the ACOG recommendation to screen for childhood sexual abuse (ACOG, 2011), the American College of Nurse Midwives' (ACNM) position statement on gender-based violence recommends routine screening for current and past violence, when best practices to ensure safety and support are in place (ACNM, 2022). Psychosocial screening (including screening for trauma history) is recommended by the Royal Australian and New Zealand College of Obstetricians and Gynaecologists (RANZCOG, 2018). The Marcé International Society is favorable toward psychosocial assessment with the proviso that skills training and clinical supervision are in place and paired with the adequacy of resources to respond to disclosures (Austin, 2014). A similar set of recommendations exists in relation to screening for IPV by the World Health Organization (WHO, 2013). Based on available evidence, the WHO does not recommend universal or routine screening for all women in healthcare settings; however, it does recommend such for antenatal care due to the "dual vulnerability of pregnancy," provided that operating procedures and training are in place, there is the availability of a private setting for the inquiry, confidentiality is ensured, and referrals are in place (WHO, 2013). Taken together, it is clear that *screening for trauma is only recommended when privacy, confidentiality, and a robust system of referrals and support are in place.* Such contextual considerations are also at the forefront in relation to routine screening for depression in the perinatal period (Reilly et al., 2020). Development of substance use is often a sequelae of childhood abuse, and perinatal organizations like ACOG (2015) recommend that routine screening for substance use disorder should be undertaken, provided it is applied equally to all people, and that provisions of respect, confidentiality, and patient autonomy are met.

Overall, current recommendations related to screening in the perinatal period are piecemeal in that they implicitly regard child abuse, IPV, perinatal mood disorders, post-traumatic stress, and substance use in pregnancy as separate and seemingly unrelated entities; however, it is likely the overall combination of these risk factors that presents the highest risk for the perinatal period (e.g., McDonald et al., 2020). This suggests the need for comprehensive psychosocial assessment that circumvents the use of multiple screening tools (e.g., Austin et al., 2013; Reilly et al., 2022). Although the decision to implement perinatal screening is influenced by recommendations from professional perinatal organizations, this may not ultimately determine whether such screening occurs. Overall, studies suggest that actual screening rates are low for child abuse, IPV, and substance use (Alhusen et al., 2022; Farrow et al., 2018; Flanagan et al., 2018; Patel et al., 2021).

Screening as Part of a Continuum of Trauma-Informed Responsivity

The identified barriers to screening and the provisos of the recommendations by professional organizations make it clear that what is needed in relation to screening is to view it as part of a continuum of trauma-informed responsivity. The ACOG underscored this with its recommendation to universally implement a trauma-informed approach across all levels of practice, including implementation of universal screening for current as well as past trauma when appropriate supportive resources are present (ACOG, 2021).

Trauma has been broadly conceptualized as an event or a series of events that are experienced as harmful by an individual and which have lasting effects (Substance Abuse and Mental Health Services Administration (SAMSHA), 2014). Being trauma-informed means realizing these effects; recognizing signs and symptoms of such, not only in clients or patients but also for their families and staff who treat them; responding by integrating such knowledge into policies, procedures, and practices; and actively seeking to resist retraumatizing individuals in clinical encounters (SAMSHA, 2014). Key principles of a trauma-informed approach include working to ensure physical and emotional *safety*, maximizing *trustworthiness through transparency* and consistency, fostering *collaboration and mutuality*, validating strengths, and fostering *empowerment, voice, choice*, promoting *peer support* and mutual self-help, and attention to *cultural, historical, and gender issues* (SAMSHA, 2014). Undergirding a trauma-informed approach is a recognition that everyone has a role to play, that being trauma-informed is not the provenance of trauma therapists exclusively, and that it is a change process that involves intentional organizational and/or individual responsiveness to new knowledge and needs (Bloom et al., 2003).

Trauma-informed principles have been translated to the perinatal period to include the examination of the promise of the perinatal caregiver-client relationship as a "holding environment" within which a sense of psychological and physical safety might be established, attention is given to common concerns of survivors of abuse in the context of perinatal healthcare, and the development of trauma-specific perinatal interventions occurs (Sperlich et al., 2017). Although trauma-informed reproductive care has been recommended as a form of "universal precautions," it is not yet a universal standard of care (Owens et al., 2021). Screening for past trauma or abuse should be seen as one step in an overall continuum of trauma-informed responsivity. This includes training and preparation on the part of the system and individuals prior to commencing screening, physically screening, offering interventions and referrals, attending to trauma-related practitioner needs as well as client needs, and evaluating care to promote quality improvement and build the clinical evidence base (Sperlich et al., 2017). It also suggests the need for integrating interprofessional collaboration with trauma-informed principles in the provision of perinatal care (Horan et al., 2022).

Screening Conditions that Foster Disclosure

Although screening is only one part of this continuum of trauma-informed responsivity, it is an important one; engaging survivors of past trauma into appropriate interventions and supports is predicated on effective screening. As such, it is important to consider what conditions foster disclosure of trauma at screening and engagement with the continuum of care. Regardless of the screening or assessment tool of choice, being ready with sensitive responses to any disclosure is paramount (see Owens et al., 2021). It is also important to ensure the screener is culturally congruent, in other words, by choosing or adapting screening instruments to meet the needs and acceptability of different cultures. For example, understanding that there are different cultural understandings of physical abuse versus physical discipline when inquiring about such (Thombs et al., 2007) and understanding that those living in contexts that include significant rates of community violence may see such exposures as normative and not connected to their present pregnancy or healthcare more broadly (Gokhale et al., 2020).

Situationally specific factors have also been shown to be important for fostering disclosures; in a study by Nguyen et al. (2019) that included administering screening for past trauma across clinic settings, participants were more likely to complete self-administered screening in examination rooms versus waiting areas, implying that privacy for the screening, even when self-administered, is likely an important consideration. A potentially more important consideration speaks to the relative level of trust that clients have for their reproductive care setting and services. A survivor may not disclose if the caregiver and system with which they are interfacing are perceived as untrustworthy. The development of trust for a trauma survivor can be fraught based on previous relationships in which boundaries were transgressed and harm done, often at the hands of someone close to them. As such, clients may be reticent to disclose to clinicians who wield power over the course of their reproductive care if they do not trust they will be met with dignity and respect. This may be further complicated if the survivor has previously disclosed in other settings, including to other healthcare providers, and the response was insensitive or experienced as re-traumatizing. Clients may have also previously experienced healthcare that included mistreatment that may have eroded trust. In a large survey of 2700 United States participants, one in six reported maltreatment experiences during their maternity care, including being shouted at, scolded, threatened, ignored, or having their requests for help refused (Vedam et al., 2019). This stresses the need for systems to critically examine their practices, procedures, and policies to align with a trauma-informed approach more closely, provide respectful care, and facilitate the development of trusting relationships between clients and care providers. Although literature related to the evaluation of projects to align perinatal practice with trauma-informed principles and practices is nascent, efforts to develop such models are underway, including the development of an integrated gynecologic and psychiatric care practice for survivors of sex trafficking and sexual violence in New York City (Ades et al., 2019).

Brief Review of Available Tools

Equally important to the context, timing, responsivity of practitioners, and availability of resources is the tool used to screen for histories of child abuse. Lewis-O'Connor et al. (2019) synthesized current practices for inquiry about trauma histories, providing an extensive overview of available tools. One of the most used is the ACEs questionnaire (Felitti et al., 1998). Although designed as a retrospective assessment for an epidemiological investigation, it is a widely accepted tool across settings (Rariden et al., 2021). In its original format of 10 questions that assess five dimensions of childhood maltreatment and household dysfunction, it is relatively expeditious to complete; however, some pose concerns regarding question composition (double- and triple-barreled questions) and the accuracy of the information collected (Mendel et al., 2021). Similarly, the Childhood Trauma Questionnaire (CTQ; Bernstein et al., 1998) is another common tool used to screen for histories of abuse that assesses five dimensions of childhood maltreatment. A bit lengthier than the ACEs questionnaire, posing some concerns regarding client burden, some regard this validated tool as the current "gold-standard" among self-reporting assessments of histories of child abuse (Schmidt et al., 2020). The CTQ is also copyrighted, making accessibility a concern for some.

A broader measure, the Antenatal Risk Questionnaire (ANRQ; Austin et al., 2013) is a tool designed to assess the psychosocial health of the pregnant person, including such things as the history of mental health conditions, relationships, social supports, recent life stressors, as well as ACEs. Reilly et al. (2022) have recently explored the validity of a revised version of the questionnaire, the ANRQ-R, in perinatal settings, found acceptable levels of concurrent and predictive validity, and concluded that it could be used effectively to identify risk factors early in pregnancy.

Another option for screening would be to look for the sequelae of the abuse rather than (or in addition to) screening for abuse itself. As such, including a brief measure of post-traumatic stress disorder (PTSD) symptomatology, such as the 5-item Primary Care PTSD (PC-PTSD-5; Prins et al., 2016) screening tool, could be used to identify those for whom referral to trauma-specific interventions might be most salient (see Chap. 3 for a more detailed exploration of PTSD and complex PTSD diagnostic criteria and their relevance to the perinatal period). Pairing assessments of histories of child abuse with current risk assessments would allow for a more thorough understanding of the circumstances of the pregnant person and more focused and timely linkages to resources.

Basic Recommendations and Precautions Across Contexts

Regardless of the choice of the screening tool, we offer some basic recommendations and precautions for applying a trauma-informed lens to screening. These include:

1. *Careful preparation and education on the part of the clinician doing the screening and the healthcare team.* This includes choosing a measure appropriate to the population, ideally one with evidence of psycho-

metric validation. It also requires familiarizing oneself with the tool and its usage, including practicing using the tool and anticipating potential responses ahead of time.

2. *Identification of optimal procedures for implementing the screening.* This includes thinking through issues of privacy, plans for ensuring confidentiality, and the adequacy of time to complete the screening, respond to any disclosures, and facilitate referrals. In tandem with screening, it may be valuable to display environmental cues such as posters for local IPV resources or support groups that might help signal to survivors that the environment is one that values assisting trauma survivors. Optimal procedures also include developing a robust and up-to-date system of referral resources so that staff conducting or reviewing screening can adequately respond with a good working knowledge of the available resources.

3. *Establishing good rapport first.* It is important to take time to establish rapport with a client before asking about past trauma. As many people have experienced abuse in the context of relationships, trust can be difficult, and survivors are looking to clinicians for authenticity and positive regard. Also, maintaining an overall tone of empathy and non-judgment is critical to fostering disclosures.

4. *Identifying any self-triggers and establishing supervision.* Screening for past abuse and/or hearing disclosures of abuse from clients can mirror experiences that clinicians themselves have had. It is important for the person doing the screening to think through how any potential disclosures might be triggering their own past trauma and for perinatal services to collectively identify how they can institute opportunities for clinicians to obtain reflective supervision that addresses any vicarious trauma they might experience, either during the screening process or during clinical encounters in general. Engaging in simple self-care practices, such as mindful breathing or grounding exercises after a disclosure, can help raise awareness of the impact of taking in such details of harm in the moment and act as a preventive strategy to the potential long-term costs of enduring disclosures, such as burnout and compassion fatigue.

5. *Develop normalizing preamble language.* Survivors may feel that they are being singled out for trauma screening. Developing a short pre-

amble might help in this regard. For instance, *"This next set of questions asks about any traumatic or adverse experiences you might have had, if you choose to share that information with us. Having experienced trauma is a very common experience. Recent research has shown that trauma may affect a person's health in a variety of ways. Because of that, we ask all of our clients about their history of trauma so that we can identify ways we might be able to help."* Note that such a preamble both normalizes the screening and provides assurance to the survivor that screening is intended to identify present-focused issues pertinent to the provision of reproductive care. It also underscores the voluntary nature of any disclosures and asserts the client's control of their voice and choice.

6. *Connecting past trauma to the present.* If a client endorses a history of trauma, clinicians can further inquire whether the client sees any specific linkages between their past trauma and the present. Machtinger et al. (2019) suggest responding with "Past traumas can sometimes continue to affect our lives and health. Do you feel like this experience continues to affect your health or well-being?" An additional follow-up question is also important to maintain the present focus: "If so, in what ways?"

7. *Addressing confidentiality.* In addition to sharing the purpose of the screening, it is important to assure the client or patient that the information they share will remain confidential. They also need to know whether there are any limits to confidentiality. For example, most clinicians have a mandatory duty to report abuse or neglect of a child or a dependent adult. A client may be concerned about who you will share this information with and may fear being judged or experiencing other negative consequences if their information were to be revealed. Therefore, the clinician should reassure the client or patient of the practice of confidentiality and inform them of any conditions under which confidentiality would be broken.

8. *Being an active listener.* Clinicians need to give the client their full attention, not interrupt, fidget, or stare at the computer screen and not the client. A good practice is to thank the client for their sharing. For some clients, this may be the first time any provider has asked them about their trauma history or the first time they have disclosed

it. Thanking the client for sharing is one simple way of acknowledging that you heard the client. *Not* saying anything at all can have the effect of silencing the client, and clinician silence could be perceived as shaming or blaming.

9. *Validate, empathize, and show support.* Try to do this in a way that does not layer the clinician's judgment on top of the situation or express pity for the person. A clinician could say things like, *"I'm sorry that happened to you,"* or *"I imagine that has been difficult for you."* Remember that showing support is not about trying to sweep away the past under a rug. Avoid suggesting that they "try not think about it," "just get over it," or "try to move on." Note, if screening is being conducted using paper or electronic screening tools in lieu of a conversation, not following up with the client could also be received as insensitive and invalidating.

10. *Right-size the response.* Try to match the client's affect around the disclosure. Some clients may indicate that they have had trauma exposures, but their trauma-related needs may be minimal. They may have a relatively easy time sharing. In this case, an introductory explanation about why trauma is being asked about, together with active listening skills, may be all that is needed. It may be enough for the client to know that although they are doing fine right now, help is available if needed. Other clients might find it much harder to share their sensitive information. If a client's body language is closed (e.g., crossed limbs or looking away), and they answer reluctantly or quietly, a response could be as simple as a sympathetic, kindly nod, or saying, *"I am so sorry about your experience. Thank you for sharing that."* If the client is more expressive, is perhaps teary or seems embarrassed, then it may make sense to add something along the lines of, *"You are certainly not alone in having experienced that. It is so common, unfortunately."* Some clients might lead with a bit of anger when being asked sensitive questions. In such instances, it might be important to restate the introductory remarks to remind the client why trauma is being asked about, and that they do not have to share anything they do not wish to. If this is the first time the client has disclosed, and particularly if abuse is current, the client may cry or share details of the traumatic exposure. Right-sizing a response in this situ-

ation will include not only thanking them for sharing, expressing empathy, and normalizing that they are not alone, but also letting them know that help is available for processing and working through their trauma, and that resources are at hand. This is particularly important for those who are disclosing about current violence. In such instances, it is important to remember what might seem somewhat counterintuitive. First, it is not appropriate to tell a person in an abusive relationship that they should leave their abuser. There may be many reasons why this is difficult or impossible. Research shows that a person is in the most danger when they leave an abusive relationship (Tjaden, 2000). Remember that although a clinician may have a mandatory duty to report current violence directed toward a child or dependent adult, an independent adult has the choice to report or seek help for their situation.

11. *Make appropriate referrals.* A carefully vetted list of referral resources must be readily available before conducting any screening. These should minimally include those for any available trauma-specific interventions and treatments appropriate for the childbearing year, substance use programs, and IPV programs.

Screening from the Perspective of the Survivor

Nascent research specifically about the perspectives of survivors regarding screening largely mirrors the above recommendations. Olsen et al. (2021) found that preferred approaches to screening included the provision of information, including the relevance of the screening and assurances regarding how the information will not be used, avoidance of re-traumatization through empathic listening and trauma-informed approaches, ensuring services are available to help before heedlessly screening, and respect for privacy and understanding that some survivors may not choose to disclose. This is underscored in qualitative research with survivors of sexual abuse during the childbearing year. Exercising control over the childbearing experience to the extent possible is viewed as promoting safety; if this is not possible, then avoidance may be employed; if these strategies do not work, then survivors feel unsafe and are vulnerable to experiencing their encounters with the birth and their providers as retraumatizing (Montgomery, 2013; Montgomery et al., 2015; Sperlich & Seng, 2008; White et al., 2016). Therefore, in all clinical interactions, it is paramount to avoid reenacting abusive scenarios.

Recommendations for Trauma Responsivity in the Absence of Screening or Disclosure

As mentioned, some survivors of child abuse may choose not to disclose to perinatal providers because they may not think it is relevant to their current care (Gokhale et al., 2020; Seng et al., 2008). A small percentage (3%) of clients in maternal-infant home visiting settings find it extremely uncomfortable to complete the ACEs, which was statistically associated with their provider's discomfort with completing the ACEs themselves (Mersky et al., 2019). Some survivors have been met with silence, shock, or dismissal during previous disclosures with providers, influencing their willingness to disclose in perinatal settings (Leeners et al., 2006). However, attuned and trauma-aware practitioners may recognize nonverbal cues during clinical interactions that may be indicators of distress, such as body tension or rapid breathing, restlessness, poor eye contact, or aggressive behavior, and can respond "as if" they are dealing with triggered trauma reactions, and work to modify care to prevent further potential retraumatization (Kuzma et al., 2020). Likewise, providers may suspect linkages to past trauma evidenced by maladaptive coping behaviors, such as substance use or disordered eating (Machtinger et al., 2019), or may intuit unspoken messages in patient requests for female members of staff or requests for planned cesarean sections (Montgomery et al., 2015). Practitioners relying solely on positive screens for child abuse may be less attuned to recognizing such cues, behaviors, and unspoken messages that indicate underlying problems or distress (Montgomery et al., 2015). This underscores the importance of providing trauma-informed and patient-centered care that validates a person's unique experience and adapts caregiving as needed.

Embodying trauma-informed principles in the perinatal period and facilitating effective screening are predicated on a perinatal workforce well-educated on the effects of trauma and its sequelae during childbearing and parenting. Such knowledge will likely be facilitative of effective and sensitive trauma inquiry. However, as Machtinger et al. (2019) have succinctly stated, "The choice of approach to inquiring about past trauma depends on the resources, expertise, and patient population of individual providers and practices" (p. 100). They recommend four basic options regarding inquiry: (1) assuming a history of trauma without asking (and offering referrals), (2) screening for impacts of past trauma rather than the trauma itself (anxiety, depression, PTSD, substance use, etc.), (3) inquiring about past trauma using open-ended questions (rather than using a formal screening tool), and 4) using a structured (and validated) tool.

Addressing Provider Trauma as a Requisite for Effective Screening

Adequacy of resources, expertise, and knowledge about the patient/client population may not be enough to effectively inquire in any of the above categories if provider trauma is not also considered. The ACOG 2011 committee opinion recommends asking about past sexual trauma in a natural, routine manner; however, this may not come naturally for a perinatal health worker who may themselves be a survivor or may just be wary of asking these sorts of sensitive questions. Instead, it is often a dynamic, complex interaction that requires education on the part of the practitioner and an acknowledgment of how trauma affects not only patients but also providers and the overall healthcare system (Stokes et al., 2017). Although there is little in the way of anticipatory guidance about conducting trauma inquiry in clinical perinatal settings, Coles and Mudaly (2010) have developed strategies and recommendations for child abuse researchers that likely have salience for clinicians as well. They underscore the importance of developing meaningful connections with their participants while at the same time acknowledging the need for role clarity and not crossing the border into providing therapy, and further acknowledge the vulnerability that researchers have for experiencing secondary traumatic stress. Strategies for minimizing such vulnerability include education, preparation, effective management of workloads, and seeking support through formal supervision (Coles & Mudaly, 2010). Establishing such strategies in perinatal workplaces could help support clinicians who are themselves survivors of childhood abuse and thereby increase the effectiveness of screening and overall provision of care. Having such supports, mechanisms, and "safe places to share" is particularly important for addressing staff trauma following critical events, which in perinatal workplaces can include maternal or infant losses (Foreman, 2014).

Summary

The reasons "why" we should screen for child abuse in the perinatal period are clear. However, barriers exist to effective screening and must be addressed. Despite barriers, many professional perinatal organizations recommend screening to identify those who are most at risk. For screening to be effective, it is optimal to view screening as part of a continuum of trauma responsivity that includes training, preparation, screening, offering referrals and interventions, and evaluating care. Instead of "why screen," the larger concern is "how we screen," taking care to consider the cultural context, timing, and setting in our choice of screening tool, and, importantly, apply a trauma-sensitive lens to screening practices across contexts, including in instances where we suspect child abuse has occurred in the absence of a disclosure. A critical component to applying such a lens is robustly addressing care provider trauma. Instead of proceeding with trauma-sensitivity, we must consider "whether to screen" when no referral resources or interventions exist. Providing adequacy of staff training and skill development regarding trauma-informed responsivity, establishing the adequacy of support and supervision for the workforce, and increasing the availability of trauma-specific perinatal interventions are aspirational goals that will necessitate a real commitment of time and financial resources to realize.

Screening for child abuse in the perinatal period must proceed in tandem with the creation, evaluation, and availability of trauma-specific interventions. Fortunately, such interventions are being created and evaluated for addressing PTSD during pregnancy (see Stevens et al., 2021) as well as for IPV (see Van Parys et al., 2014), and for perinatal depression resulting from childhood trauma (see Reuveni et al., 2021), although more research is needed to evaluate their effectiveness. There is also a lack of interventions that specifically address the needs of fathers with child abuse trauma, same-sex couples, and aboriginal families (Chamberlain et al., 2019). In conclusion, it is time to fully commit to the transformational undertaking of establishing trauma-informed care in perinatal spaces. Those who have suffered much deserve nothing less.

References

Ades, V., Wu, S. X., Rabinowitz, E., Bach, S. C., Goddard, B., Ayala, S. P., & Greene, J. (2019). An integrated, trauma-informed care model for female survivors of sexual violence: The engage, motivate, protect, organize, self-worth, educate, respect (EMPOWER) clinic. *Obstetrics & Gynecology, 133*(4), 803–809. https://doi.org/10.1097/AOG.0000000000003186

Alhusen, J. L., Lyons, G., Laughon, K., & Hughes, R. B. (2022). Intimate partner violence during the perinatal period by disability status: Findings from a United States population-based analysis. *Journal of Advanced Nursing, 00*, 1–10. https://doi.org/10.1111/jan.15340

American College of Nurse-Midwives (ACNM). (2022). *Position statement: Gender-based violence.* https://www.midwife.org/acnm/files/acnmlibrary-data/uploadfilename/000000000091/FINAL_GENDER%20BASED%20VIOLENCE_04112022.pdf

American College of Obstetricians and Gynecologists. (2015). Committee opinion no. 633: Alcohol abuse and other substance use disorders: Ethical issues in obstetric and gynecologic practice. *Obstetrics and Gynecology, 125*(6), 1529–1537. https://doi.org/10.1097/01.AOG.0000466371.86393.9b

American College of Obstetricians and Gynecologists, & Committee on Health Care for Underserved Women. (2021). Caring for patients who have experienced trauma: ACOG Committee Opinion, number 825. *Obstetrics and Gynecology, 137*(4), e94–e99.

American College of Obstetricians and Gynecologists (ACOG). (2011). Adult manifestations of childhood sexual abuse. Committee Opinion No. 498.

Obstetrics & Gynecology, 118, 392–395. https://doi.org/10.1097/ AOG.0B013E31822C994D

Atzl, V. M., Narayan, A. J., Rivera, L. M., & Lieberman, A. F. (2019). Adverse childhood experiences and prenatal mental health: Type of ACEs and age of maltreatment onset. *Journal of Family Psychology, 33*(3), 304–314. https:// doi.org/10.1037/fam0000510

Austin, M. P., Colton, J., Priest, S., Reilly, N., & Hadzi-Pavolvic. (2013). The Antenatal Risk Questionnaire (ANQR): Acceptability and use for psychosocial risk assessment in the maternity setting. *Women & Birth, 26*(1), 17–25. https://doi.org/10.1016/j.wombi.2011.06.002

Austin, M. P., & Marcé Society Position Statement Advisory Committee. (2014). Marcé International Society position statement on psychosocial assessment and depression screening in perinatal women. *Best Practice & Research Clinical Obstetrics & Gynaecology, 28*(1), 179–187. https://doi. org/10.1016/j.bpobgyn.2013.08.016

Bernstein, D. P., Fink, L., Handelsman, L., & Foote, J. (1998). Childhood trauma questionnaire. In *Assessment of family violence: A handbook for researchers and practitioners.* American Psychological Association.

Bloom, S. L., Bennington-Davis, M., Farragher, B., McCorkle, D., Nice-Martini, K., & Wellbank, K. (2003). Multiple opportunities for creating sanctuary. *Psychiatric Quarterly, 74,* 173–190. https://doi.org/10.1023/ a:1021359828022

Carroll, M., Downes, C., Gill, A., Monahan, M., Nagle, U., Madden, D., & Higgins, A. (2018). Knowledge, confidence, skills and practices among midwives in the Republic of Ireland in relation to perinatal mental health care: The mind mothers study. *Midwifery, 64,* 29–37. https://doi.org/10.1016/j. midw.2018.05.006

Chamberlain, C., Gee, G., Harfield, S., Campbell, S., Brennan, S., Clark, Y., et al. (2019). Parenting after a history of childhood maltreatment: A scoping review and map of evidence in the perinatal period. *PLoS One, 14*(3), e0213460. https://doi.org/10.1371/journal.pone.0213460

Coles, J., & Mudaly, N. (2010). Staying safe: Strategies for qualitative child abuse researchers. *Child Abuse Review, 19*(1), 56–69. https://doi. org/10.1002/car.1080

Docherty, A., Najjar, R., Combs, S., Woolley, R., & Stoyles, S. (2020). Postpartum depression screening in the first year: A cross-sectional provider analysis in Oregon. *Journal of the American Association of Nurse Practitioners, 32*(4), 308–315. https://doi.org/10.1097/JXX.0000000000000250

Farrow, V. A., Bosch, J., Crawford, J. N., Snead, C., & Schulkin, J. (2018). Screening for history of childhood abuse: Beliefs, practice patterns, and barriers among obstetrician-gynecologists. *Women's Health Issues, 28*(6), 559–568. https://doi.org/10.1016/j.whi.2018.09.001

Felitti, V. J., Anda, R. F., Nordenberg, D., Williamson, D. F., Spitz, A. M., Edwards, V., Koss, M. P., & Marks, J. S. (1998). Relationship of childhood abuse and household dysfunction to many of the leading causes of death in adult: The adverse childhood experiences (ACE) study. *American Journal of Preventive Medicine, 14*(4), 245–258. https://doi.org/10.1016/S0749-3797(98)00017-8

Finkelhor, D. (2018). Screening for adverse childhood experiences (ACEs): Cautions and suggestions. *Child Abuse & Neglect, 85*, 174–179. https://doi.org/10.1016/j.chiabu.2017.07.016

Flanagan, T., Alabaster, A., McCaw, B., Stoller, N., Watson, C., & Young-Wolff, K. C. (2018). Feasibility and acceptability of screening for adverse childhood experiences in prenatal care. *Journal of Women's Health, 27*(7), 903–911. https://doi.org/10.1089/jwh.2017.6649

Foreman, S. (2014). Developing a process to support perinatal nurses after a critical event. *Nursing for Women's Health, 18*(1), 61–65. https://doi.org/10.1111/1751-486X.12094

Gokhale, P., Young, M. R., Williams, M. N., Reid, S. N., Tom, L. S., O'Brian, C. A., & Simon, M. A. (2020). Refining trauma-informed perinatal care for urban prenatal care patients with multiple lifetime traumatic exposures: A qualitative study. *Journal of Midwifery & Women's Health, 65*(2), 224–230. https://doi.org/10.1111/jmwh.13063

Horan, H., Ryu, J., Stone, J., & Thurston, L. (2022). Healing trauma with interprofessional collaboration and trauma-informed perinatal care: A qualitative case study. *Birth, 50*, 1–10. https://doi.org/10.1111/birt.12672

Hutchens, B. F., Kearney, J., & Kennedy, H. P. (2017). Survivors of child maltreatment and postpartum depression: An integrative review. *Journal of Midwifery & Women's Health, 62*(6), 706–722. https://doi.org/10.1111/jmwh.12680

Kuzma, E. K., Pardee, M., & Morgan, A. (2020). Implementing patient-centered trauma-informed care for the perinatal nurse. *The Journal of Perinatal & Neonatal Nursing, 34*(4), E23–E31. https://doi.org/10.1097/JPN.0000000000000520

Lee, A., Coles, J., Lee, S. J., & Kulkarni, J. (2012). Women survivors of child abuse: Don't ask, don't tell. *Australian Family Physician, 41*(11), 903–906. https://doi.org/10.3316/informit.896943579195322

Leeners, B., Richter-Appelt, H., Imthurn, B., & Rath, W. (2006). Influence of childhood sexual abuse on pregnancy, delivery, and the early postpartum period in adult women. *Journal of Psychosomatic Research, 61*(2), 139–151. https://doi.org/10.1016/j.jpsychores.2005.11.006

Leeners, B., Stiller, R., Block, E., Görres, G., & Rath, W. (2010). Pregnancy complications in women with childhood sexual abuse experiences. *Journal of Psychosomatic Research, 69*(5), 503–510. https://doi.org/10.1016/j.jpsychores.2010.04.017

Lewis-O'Connor, A., Warren, A., Lee, J. V., Levy-Carrick, N., Grossman, S., Chadwick, M., Stoklosa, H., & Rittenberg, E. (2019). The state of the science on trauma inquiry. *Women's Health, 15*, 1745506519861234. https://doi.org/10.1177/1745506519861234

Machtinger, E. L., Davis, K. B., Kimberg, L. S., Khanna, N., Cuca, Y. P., Dawson-Rose, C., Shumway, M., Campbell, J., Lewis-O'Connor, A., Blake, M., Blanch, A., & McCaw, B. (2019). From treatment to healing: Inquiry and response to recent and past trauma in adult health care. *Women's Health Issues, 29*(2), 97–102. https://doi.org/10.1016/j.whi.2018.11.003

Maunder, R. G., Hunter, J. J., Tannenbaum, D. W., Le, T. L., & Lay, C. (2020). Physicians' knowledge and practices regarding screening adult patients for adverse childhood experiences: A survey. *BMC Health Services Research, 20*(1), 1–5. https://doi.org/10.1186/s12913-020-05124-6

McDonald, L. R., Antoine, D. G., Liao, C., Lee, A., Wahab, M., & Coleman, J. S. (2020). Syndemic of lifetime mental illness, substance use disorders, and trauma and their association with adverse perinatal outcomes. *Journal of Interpersonal Violence, 35*(1–2), 476–495. https://doi.org/10.1177/0886260516685708

McLennan, J. D., McTavish, J. R., & MacMillan, H. L. (2020). Routine screening of ACEs: Should we or shouldn't we? In *Adverse childhood experiences* (pp. 145–159). Academic Press.

Mendel, W., Sperlich, M., & Fava, N. (2021). "Is there anything else you would like me to know?": Applying a trauma-informed approach to the administration of the Adverse Childhood Experiences (ACE) questionnaire. *Journal of Community Psychology, 49*, 1079–1099. https://doi.org/10.1002/jcop.22562

Mersky, J. P., Lee, C. T. P., & Gilbert, R. M. (2019). Client and provider discomfort with an adverse childhood experiences survey. *American Journal of Preventive Medicine, 57*(2), e51–e58. https://doi.org/10.1016/j.amepre.2019.02.026

Millar, H. C., Lorber, S., Vandermorris, A., Thompson, G., Thompson, M., Allen, L., Aggarwal, A., & Spitzer, R. F. (2021). "No, you need to explain what you are doing": Obstetric care experiences and preferences of adolescent mothers with a history of childhood trauma. *Journal of Pediatric and Adolescent Gynecology, 34*(4), 538–545. https://doi.org/10.1016/j.jpag.2021.01.006

Montgomery, E. (2013). Feeling safe: A metasynthesis of the maternity care needs of women who were sexually abused in childhood. *Birth, 40*(2), 88–95. https://doi.org/10.1111/birt.12043

Montgomery, E., Pope, C., & Rogers, J. (2015). A feminist narrative study of the maternity care experiences of women who were sexually abused in childhood. *Midwifery, 31*(1), 54–60. https://doi.org/10.1016/j.midw.2014.05.010

Muzik, M., Bocknek, E. L., Broderick, A., Richardson, P., Rosenblum, K. L., Thelen, K., & Seng, J. S. (2013). Mother-infant bonding impairment across the first 6 months postpartum: The primacy of psychopathology in women with childhood abuse and neglect histories. *Archives of Women's Mental Health, 16*(1), 29–38. https://doi.org/10.1007/s00737-012-0312-0

Newcomb, M. D., & Locke, T. F. (2001). Intergenerational cycle of maltreatment: A popular concept obscured by methodological limitations. *Child Abuse & Neglect, 25*(9), 1219–1240. https://doi.org/10.1016/S0145-2134(01)00267-8

Nguyen, M. W., Heberlein, E., Covington-Kolb, S., Gerstner, A. M., Gaspard, A., & Eichelberger, K. Y. (2019). Assessing adverse childhood experiences during pregnancy: Evidence toward a best practice. *American Journal of Perinatology Reports, 9*(01), e54–e59. https://doi.org/10.1055/s-0039-1683407

Olsen, J. M., Galloway, E. G., & Guthman, P. L. (2021). Exploring women's perspectives on prenatal screening for adverse childhood experiences. *Public Health Nursing, 38*(6), 997–1008. https://doi.org/10.1111/phn.12956

Owens, L., Terrell, S., Low, L. K., Loder, C., Rhizal, D., Scheiman, L., & Seng, J. (2021). Universal precautions: The case for consistently trauma-informed reproductive healthcare. *American Journal of Obstetrics and Gynecology, 226*(5), 671–677. https://doi.org/10.1016/j.ajog.2021.08.012

Patel, E., Bandara, S., Saloner, B., Stuart, E. A., Goodman, D., Terplan, M., McCourt, A., White, S., & McGinty, E. E. (2021). Heterogeneity in prenatal substance use screening despite universal screening recommendations: Findings from the Pregnancy Risk Assessment Monitoring System, 2016–2018. *American Journal of Obstetrics & Gynecology MFM, 3*(5), 100419. https://doi.org/10.1016/j.ajogmf.2021.100419

Prins, A., Bovin, M. J., Smolenski, D. J., Marx, B. P., Kimerling, R., Jenkins-Guarnieri, M. A., Kaloupek, D. G., Schnurr, P., Kaiser, A. P., Leyva, Y. E., & Tiet, Q. Q. (2016). The primary care PTSD screen for DSM-5 (PC-PTSD-5): Development and evaluation within a veteran primary care sample. *Journal of*

General Internal Medicine, 31(10), 1206–1211. https://doi.org/10.1007/s11606-016-3703-5

RANZCOG. (2018). *Mental Health Care in the perinatal period* (C-Obs 48).

Rariden, C., SmithBattle, L., Yoo, J. H., Cibulka, N., & Loman, D. (2021). Screening for adverse childhood experiences: Literature review and practice implications. *The Journal for Nurse Practitioners, 17*(1), 98–104. https://doi.org/10.1016/j.nurpra.2020.08.002

Reilly, N., Hadzi-Pavolvic, D., Loxton, D., Black, E., Mule, V., & Austin, M. P. (2022). Supporting routine psychosocial assessment in the perinatal period: The concurrent and predictive validity of the Antenatal Risk Questionnaire-Revised. *Women and Birth, 35*(2), e118–e124. https://doi.org/10.1016/j.wombi.2021.04.003

Reilly, N., Kingston, D., Loxton, D., Talcevska, K., & Austin, M. P. (2020). A narrative review of studies addressing the clinical effectiveness of perinatal depression screening programs. *Women and Birth, 33*(1), 51–59. https://doi.org/10.1016/j.wombi.2019.03.004

Reuveni, I., Lauria, M., Monk, C., & Werner, E. (2021). The impact of childhood trauma on psychological interventions for depression during pregnancy and postpartum: A systematic review. *Archives of Women's Mental Health, 24*(3), 367–380. https://doi.org/10.1007/s00737-020-01066-4

Schmidt, M. R., Narayan, A., Atzl, V. M., Rivera, L. M., & Lieberman, A. F. (2020). Childhood maltreatment on the Adverse Childhood Experiences (ACEs) scale versus the Childhood Trauma Questionnaire (CTQ) in a perinatal sample. *Journal of Aggression, Maltreatment & Trauma, 29*(1), 38–56. https://doi.org/10.1080/10926771.2018.1524806

Seng, J., Sperlich, M., & Kane Low, L. (2008). Mental health, demographic, and risk behavior profiles of pregnant survivors of childhood and adult abuse. *Journal of Midwifery & Women's Health, 53*(6), 511–521. https://doi.org/10.1016/j.jmwh.2008.04.013

Seng, J. S., Kane Low, L., Sperlich, M., Ronis, D., & Liberzon, I. (2011). Posttraumatic stress disorder, child abuse history, birthweight and gestational age: A prospective cohort study. *BJOG: British Journal of Obstetrics and Gynaecology, 118*(11), 1329–1339. https://doi.org/10.1111/j.1471-0528.2011

Seng, J. S., Kane Low, L. M., Sperlich, M. I., Ronis, D. L., & Liberzon, I. (2009). Prevalence, trauma history and risk for PTSD among nulliparous women in maternity care. *Obstetrics & Gynecology, 114*(4), 839–847. https://doi.org/10.1097/AOG.0b013e181b8f8a2

Seng, J. S., Sperlich, M., Kane Low, L., Ronis, D. L., Muzik, M., & Liberzon, I. (2013). Child abuse history, posttraumatic stress disorder, postpartum mental health, and bonding: A prospective cohort study. *Journal of Midwifery & Women's Health*, *58*(1), 57–68. https://doi.org/10.1111/j.1542-2011.2012.00237.x

Souch, A. J., Jones, I. R., Shelton, K. H., & Waters, C. S. (2022). Maternal childhood maltreatment and perinatal outcomes: A systematic review. *Journal of Affective Disorders*, *302*(1), 139–159. https://doi.org/10.1016/j.jad.2022.01.062

Sperlich, M., Seng, J., Yang, L., Taylor, J., & Bradbury-Jones, C. (2017). Integrating trauma-informed care into midwifery practice: Conceptual and practical issues. *Journal of Midwifery & Women's Health*, *62*(6), 661–672. https://doi.org/10.1111/jmwh.12674

Sperlich, M., & Seng, J. S. (2008). *Survivor moms: Women's stories of birthing, mothering and healing after sexual abuse*. Motherbaby Press.

Stevens, N. R., Miller, M. L., Puetz, A. K., Padin, A. C., Adams, N., & Meyer, D. J. (2021). Psychological intervention and treatment for posttraumatic stress disorder during pregnancy: A systematic review and call to action. *Journal of Traumatic Stress, 34*(3), 575–585. https://doi.org/10.1002/jts.22641

Stokes, Y., Jacob, J.-D., Gifford, W., Squires, J., & Vandyk, A. (2017). Exploring nurses' knowledge and experiences related to trauma-informed care. *Global Qualitative Nursing Research*, *4*, 2333393617734510. https://doi.org/10.1177/2333393617734510

Substance Abuse and Mental Health Services Administration. (2014). *SAMHSA's concept of trauma and guidance for a trauma-informed approach* (HHS Publication No. (SMA) 14-4884). U.S. Department of Health and Human Services. https://ncsacw.samhsa.gov/userfiles/files/SAMHSA_Trauma.pdf

Thackeray, J., Stelzner, S., Downs, S. M., & Miller, C. (2007). Screening for intimate partner violence: The impact of screener and screening environment on victim comfort. *Journal of Interpersonal Violence, 22*(6), 659–670. https://doi.org/10.1177/0886260507300206

Thombs, B. D., Bennett, W., Ziegelstein, R. C., Bernstein, D. P., Scher, C. D., & Forde, D. R. (2007). Cultural sensitivity in screening adults for a history of childhood abuse: Evidence from a community sample. *Journal of General Internal Medicine, 22*(3), 368–373. https://doi.org/10.1007/s11606-006-0026-y

Tjaden, P. G. (2000). *Extent, nature, and consequences of intimate partner violence*. US Department of Justice, Office of Justice Programs, National Institute of Justice.

Van Parys, A. S., Verhamme, A., Temmerman, M., & Verstraelen, H. (2014). Intimate partner violence and pregnancy: A systematic review of interventions. *PLoS One, 9*(1), e85084. https://doi.org/10.1371/journal.pone.0085084

Vedam, S., Stoll, K., Taiwo, T. K., Rubashkin, N., Cheyney, M., Strauss, N., et al. (2019). The giving voice to mothers study: Inequity and mistreatment during pregnancy and childbirth in the United States. *Reproductive Health, 16*(1), 1–18. https://doi.org/10.1186/s12978-019-0729-2

Watson, K., White, C., Hall, H., & Hewitt, A. (2021). Women's experiences of birth trauma: A scoping review. *Women and Birth, 34*(5), 417–424. https://doi.org/10.1016/j.wombi.2020.09.016

White, A., Danis, M., & Gillece, J. (2016). Abuse survivor perspectives on trauma inquiry in obstetrical practice. *Archives of Women's Mental Health, 19*(2), 423–427. https://doi.org/10.1007/s00737-015-0547-7

World Health Organization. (2013). *Responding to intimate partner violence and sexual violence against women: WHO clinical and policy guidelines.* World Health Organization.

Yu, M., & Sampson, M. (2019). Pediatrician attitudes and practices regarding postpartum depression screening: Training and interprofessional collaboration needed. *Journal of Interprofessional Education & Practice, 15*, 1–4. https://doi.org/10.1016/j.xjep.2018.12.005

8

Building Resilience in the Perinatal Period for Survivors of Childhood Adversity

Nicole Racine ⓘ, Teresa E. Killam, Julianna Park, and Sheri Madigan

Abstract Exposure to abuse in childhood can have long-term implications for physical and mental health across the life course, including the perinatal period. However, bourgeoning research demonstrates that child abuse experiences are far from deterministic, with several factors contributing to resilience in the face of adversity. This chapter provides an overview of resilience science as it relates to the impact of child abuse on health and mental health in pregnancy and the postpartum period. Using a bioecological framework, we review the scientific literature on promotive and protective factors across the social ecology, including the individual level

N. Racine (✉)
University of Ottawa, Children's Hospital of Eastern Ontario,
Ottawa, ON, Canada
e-mail: nracine2@uottawa.ca

T. E. Killam
Riley Park Maternity Clinic, University of Calgary, Calgary, AB, Canada

J. Park • S. Madigan
University of Calgary, Calgary, AB, Canada

(e.g., coping skills), family level (e.g., partner support), community level (e.g., social support from neighbors, colleagues, or friends), and system level (e.g., the built environment) associated with resilience in pregnant individuals with experiences of child abuse. We provide examples of programs and interventions at diverse levels of the social ecology that promote resilience in pregnancy and the postpartum. Finally, we provide directions for future research and practice.

Keywords Resilience • Child abuse • Adverse childhood experience • Perinatal • Woman • Pregnancy

Nearly one-third of adults report exposure to some form of abuse in their childhood (Afifi et al., 2014). Left unaddressed, exposure to child abuse may increase the risk of physical and mental health challenges across the life span (Hughes et al., 2017). One life course stage that may be particularly impacted by the effects of child abuse is the perinatal period (Hudziak, 2018). Specifically, child abuse has been associated with an increased risk of pregnancy complications (Kern et al., 2022a; Kern et al., 2022b; Leeners et al., 2010) and poor birth outcomes (Mersky & Lee, 2019; Miller et al., 2021; Smith et al., 2016). Recently, research is moving beyond the consideration of child abuse explicitly to consider other forms of adversity in childhood, including neglect and household dysfunction, such as having a family member with substance use or severe mental health difficulties. The accumulation of adverse childhood experiences (ACEs), including exposure to abuse, neglect, and household dysfunction, is associated with poor physical (Olsen, 2018) and mental health (Cooke et al., 2021) in the perinatal period. Increasing evidence also demonstrates that the impacts of ACEs are intergenerational (Cooke et al., 2021). That is, maternal exposure to childhood abuse can be transmitted to offspring via biological and psychosocial pathways that occur in the pregnancy and postpartum (Madigan et al., 2017; Racine et al., 2018b). For example, children of mothers with high levels of ACEs are twice as likely to be diagnosed with a developmental delay than children of mothers exposed to low levels of ACEs (Folger et al., 2018). Although ACEs demonstrate a long reach into the perinatal period, negative outcomes for women with childhood abuse histories are far from universal (Young-Wolff et al., 2019). Many women demonstrate positive adaptation or better than expected outcomes (i.e., resilience) despite their childhood histories of abuse.

Given the pernicious influence of ACEs on both maternal and child health outcomes, building understanding of the factors that can promote resilience despite these exposures is critical. Specifically, understanding "when" and "for whom" the negative shadow of ACEs can be disrupted is needed to inform policy and practice. This chapter aims to provide a comprehensive overview of theories of resilience, describes psychosocial and biological factors that may contribute to resilience in the perinatal period for women exposed to abuse and adversity, and identifies current interventions and resilience promoting strategies that have been shown to be efficacious for perinatal women with histories of child abuse and adversity. We conclude this chapter with implications for practice and future directions for the field.

Overview of Resilience Science

Resilience science provides important theoretical underpinnings for understanding how better than expected outcomes can occur in the perinatal period for women exposed to abuse in childhood. Resilience refers to the process by which adaptive outcomes (e.g., good mental health in pregnancy) occur despite risk factors (e.g., a history of childhood sexual abuse). Risk factors are defined as threats to maternal well-being that can result in poor or negative outcomes, such as health complications or psychopathology (Masten, 2013).

In contrast, protective factors (e.g., social support, Masten, 2013) mitigate poor outcomes in the presence of risk. Key theorists in resilience science have hypothesized that risk and protective factors can exist at different levels of women's social ecology (individual, family, or community levels) (Masten, 2021). The individual level refers to protective factors that are specific to one person, such as coping skills. Protective factors at the family level are those that exist within and among members of the family or for the family as whole, such as marital satisfaction or effective co-parenting. Factors at the community level are those that exist outside the family unit, such as social support, but have an influence on both the family and the individuals within the family. Protective factors alter the association between child abuse and maternal mental health in pregnancy, leading to a resilient or improved outcome. In contrast to protective factors that modify the association between exposure to risk and an outcome, promotive factors positively affect outcomes regardless of risk exposure (Narayan et al., 2021). For example, social support leads to positive outcomes for all individuals, regardless of abuse exposure. Resilience science provides important models that can be tested to understand the process by which risk and protective factors exert their influence.

In addition to resilience science, differential susceptibility theory (Belsky & Pluess, 2009) can also help explain why some exposed to adversity in childhood experience poor perinatal outcomes, while others do not. Differential susceptibility theory purports that some individuals are highly sensitive to their environments for better *and* for worse. Women who are most impacted by negative or abusive environments may also stand to benefit most from enriching and supportive environments during pregnancy and postpartum. Women who are more temperamentally sensitive or have a genetic predisposition to mental health difficulties may be more susceptible. Thus, differential susceptibility theory sets the foundation for understanding "when" and "for whom" positive outcomes can be achieved, despite adverse experiences in childhood. A detailed discussion of differential susceptibility theory can be found in Chap. 2.

Promotive and Protective Factors in the Perinatal Period Following Child Abuse

Protective and promotive factors play a vital role in resilience during the perinatal period (Xuemei et al., 2019). Protective effects vary depending on the risk level of the individual, having greater influence at higher risk or adversity levels. In contrast, promotive effects are predictors of improved well-being independent of risk level, influencing all risk levels (Masten, 2021). The bioecological model of resilience considers how promotive and protective factors exist at various levels of the social ecology, including the individual level (e.g., coping skills), family level (e.g., partner support), community level (e.g., social support from neighbors, colleagues, or friends), and system level (e.g., the built environment) (Masten, 2021; Ungar et al., 2013). Importantly, the bioecological model of resilience stresses that resilience is not an individual trait or characteristic but involves the collective resources available to support individuals who exist within a larger system (Ungar et al., 2013). Next, we discuss promotive and protective factors associated with resilience in pregnancy and postpartum for individuals exposed to abuse in childhood.

Individual-Level Factors

Individual-level protective and promotive factors, such as self-esteem, a positive attributional style (i.e., tending to view things as positive rather than negative), and individual coping ability (i.e., ability to manage stressful situations), have been shown to be associated with improved maternal mental health during the perinatal period (Atzl et al., 2019; Xuemei et al., 2019). Self-esteem and positive attributional style have been shown to play a promotive role, being directly associated with decreased depressive symptoms and parental stress during the perinatal period (Leigh & Milgrom, 2008). Comparatively, coping ability has been shown to play a protective role, moderating the association between experience of childhood maltreatment and maternal post-traumatic stress disorder (PTSD) and depression symptoms (Sexton et al., 2015), as well as pregnancy-related anxiety (Brunton et al., 2022). Mothers with a higher perceived ability to adapt to change and recover from hardship had attenuated associations between childhood exposure to household dysfunction and post-traumatic stress symptoms in the perinatal period (Osofsky et al., 2021). Taken together, although adaptive outcomes for women exposed to abuse in childhood are multi-determined, individual skills such as increasing self-esteem and coping strategies appear to have positive implications, particularly for maternal mental health.

Family-Level Factors

Research on family-level protective factors in the perinatal period has primarily focused on two key areas: an individual's positive childhood experiences in her family of origin, such as positive parenting relationships and perceived safety and security (Atzl et al., 2019), and her experiences of support from her current identified partner and family (Racine et al., 2019). Several studies have suggested that positive childhood experiences play a protective role during the perinatal period, with positive childhood experiences being associated with improved maternal mental health, specifically decreased symptoms of PTSD and depression among women who have experienced childhood adversity (Chung et al., 2008; Narayan et al., 2018). Considering these findings, understanding how positive childhood experiences support perinatal resilience for women who have experienced childhood adversity is an important area of further research.

Partner support in pregnancy and postpartum has also been identified as an important protective factor. Research has shown that partner support is associated with reductions in maternal stress and anxiety across the pregnancy and postpartum (Racine et al., 2019). In the context of ACEs, Thomas et al. (2018) showed that partner support moderated the association between exposure to maternal ACEs and HPA axis function (i.e., biological response to stress), indicating that high levels of support from a partner are successful in dampening the association between ACEs and maternal stress responses in pregnancy. The protective effect of partner support has also been shown to be intergenerational—the positive association between ACEs and abnormal size at birth (i.e., ratio of head circumference to weight at birth) was dampened by high levels of partner support (Appleton et al., 2019). Having safe, stable, and nurturing relationships with a partner has also been shown to be a protective factor for disrupting the intergenerational transmission of maltreatment—individuals who experience safe relationships are less likely to perpetuate maltreatment themselves (Thornberry et al., 2013). Thus, encouraging partners to be socially supportive during pregnancy and postpartum may be an important prevention and intervention target.

Community-Level and System-Level Factors

Both community-level and system-level protective and promotive factors can play an important role in resilience during the perinatal period. Community-level protective and promotive factors are the social networks that shape the quality of relationships and social support available during the perinatal period. System-level protective and promotive factors are the cultural and environmental backdrop that individual-level, family-level, and community-level factors exist on. System-level factors may include cultural obligations, laws, and the built environment (Ungar et al., 2013). Below we summarize evidence for two community-level and system-level factors (i.e., community social support and neighborhood conditions) and how they can promote adaptive outcomes in the perinatal period for women with child abuse histories.

Social support, including support that is provided outside the family, such as tangible, emotional, and affective support, has been shown to be an important protective factor in mitigating anxiety and depression during the perinatal period for individuals exposed to abuse and maltreatment in childhood (Brunton et al., 2022). Social support has continued to play an important promotive role during the COVID-19 pandemic, with higher levels of perceived social support associated with lower symptoms of depression and anxiety in pregnant individuals (Lebel et al., 2020). Social support has also been shown to play a key role in disrupting the intergenerational transmission of risk in pregnancy, which is hypothesized to have cascading effects on child outcomes (Racine et al., 2018a; Thomas et al., 2018). Specifically, social support during the perinatal period moderated the association between ACEs and pregnancy complications, such that mothers who experienced ACEs had significantly lower pregnancy complications when they had higher levels of perceived social support in their lives than those who had low levels of social support (Racine et al., 2018a). It is critical to emphasize that support, even when provided outside the immediate family, can promote resilience in mothers.

The characteristics of the neighborhoods and environments where people live also can be important drivers of resilience in the face of adversity. For example, neighborhood collective efficacy (i.e., the likelihood that members of a neighborhood will act to help, are cohesive with others, and that members of the neighborhood can be trusted) moderated the association between maternal ACEs and marital conflict in a longitudinal sample of socio-demographically diverse mothers (Madigan et al., 2016). That is, resources outside the family, such as feelings of security, trust of others, and feeling connected to others, were protective against the effects of early adversity on marital discord. The availability of gyms and recreation areas as well as the walkability of a neighborhood has been associated with increased physical activity during pregnancy (Kershaw et al., 2021) and lower levels of pregnancy complications (Vinikoor-Imler et al., 2011). Although no studies to date have examined aspects of the built environment as protective against the negative effects of child abuse, the promotive effects of the built environment for maternal and infant health suggest this is a fruitful direction for future research.

Practices and Interventions that Promote Resilience in the Perinatal Period

In addition to the promotive and protective factors identified in the research literature, there is growing evidence for practices and interventions delivered at various levels of the social ecology that promote adaptive outcomes in individuals with histories of child abuse. Although some interventions target individual functioning and well-being, others are delivered at the community level, or target change within a healthcare system. That is, although some individuals may need or benefit from targeted individual support related to experiences of abuse in childhood, others may benefit from universal approaches that are available to all pregnant and parenting people. Thus, a stepped approach to support whereby everyone gets the appropriate level of support based on their needs will be most effective. Additionally, a recent review suggests that interventions that address the negative outcomes associated with maternal child abuse exposure should be strength-based, multi-systemic, and developmental in nature (Howell et al., 2021). Specifically, multi-systemic approaches work across systems (e.g., social services, medical). Developmental approaches consider the individual's developmental stage (e.g., adolescence versus adulthood). We briefly describe promising, evidence-based interventions for improving health and mental health outcomes among perinatal individuals with abuse histories.

Individual-Level Interventions

Individual-level interventions are primarily designed to increase the individual coping skills or resources of mothers with abuse histories. Two well-established interventions are the Nurse-Family Partnership (NFP) (Olds, 2006) and the Survivor Moms' Companion (SMC) (Sperlich & Seng, 2018). The NFP was one of the first home-visiting interventions to be offered in pregnancy that has demonstrated a high level of effectiveness in improving maternal mental health outcomes, child outcomes, and the prevention of child maltreatment. Through the provision of public health nurses who provide support in family planning, perinatal care, and parenting and life skill development (e.g., caring for a baby, submitting a resume, or looking for a job) through weekly appointments up to the child's second birthday, the NFP helps break the cycle of risk that can persist for individuals with histories of child abuse, ultimately leading to more adaptive outcomes for both mothers and their children (Kitzman et al., 2000; Olds et al., 1986).

The SMC is designed to promote adaptive maternal health, mental health, and parenting outcomes among those with histories of abuse. It is a weekly group that is offered over six weeks, with 2.5-hour sessions by a provider (e.g., counselor, social worker) who has been trained in the model. The intervention is delivered as a group-based intervention and provides individuals with skills for managing strong emotions, PTSD symptoms, as well as psychoeducation about the impacts of abuse and trauma. The SMC has been shown to reduce postpartum psychological distress symptoms and improve the mother-child relationship (Rowe et al., 2014). There are many hypothesized mechanisms via which SMC leads to improved outcomes for women with histories of abuse, including social support from peers, an increased understanding of trauma, and developing coping skills related to PTSD. Another group-based intervention delivered prenatally, CenteringPregnancy, may also mitigate the negative impact of child abuse on maternal outcomes, particularly postpartum depression, by increasing social support during pregnancy (Liu et al., 2021). It is a 10-session intervention, with each session lasting two hours. Although CenteringPregnancy was not specifically designed with experiences of childhood trauma in mind, the group-based pre- and postnatal care has been associated with better postpartum mental health outcomes more broadly (Buultjens et al., 2021).

Another example of the development of a recent program for pregnant individuals exposed to childhood trauma is the STEP program (Berthelot et al., 2021). The STEP program involves eight or nine sessions and is designed to be provided by two facilitators to four to six individuals. The program is trauma-informed and designed to help participants process their feelings related to becoming a mother, emotional experiences related to their past, as well as strategies for moving forward and looking ahead. There is preliminary acceptability and satisfaction as well as decreases in psychological distress shown among pregnant individuals exposed to childhood trauma (Berthelot et al., 2021). Programs targeting poor health and mental health outcomes in the aftermath of childhood trauma can improve outcomes and promote resilience.

Community-Level Interventions

In addition to formal interventions that provide psychoeducation and help build skills for women with histories of child abuse, there are also programs provided within the community that can promote resilience in the perinatal period for women with trauma histories. For example, the Pacific Postpartum Support Society is a nonprofit organization in British Columbia, Canada, that offers a suite of support to postpartum mothers using a peer support model (Handford, 2011). An important active ingredient in community-level support is the social support provided by other women with lived experiences of mental health difficulties in pregnancy and postpartum. Support that is community-based and facilitated by community members may also enhance willingness and comfort to participate, particularly for members of marginalized groups who have historically experienced discrimination and systemic racism in the health-care system (Maxwell et al., 2019). For example, a meta-interpretive synthesis of qualitative studies exploring the postpartum experiences of marginalized women found that these women were less likely to disclose their challenges to healthcare providers for fear of being judged or having their children taken away (Maxwell et al., 2019). Thus, services and support provided within communities and by trusted community members have the potential for greater reach in bolstering postpartum mental health outcomes.

Another important consideration for approaches and interventions associated with resilience in the perinatal period for women with childhood abuse histories is whether this support can address the needs of diverse populations and is culturally competent or attuned to differences across cultures. For example, a recent review of postpartum depression interventions for immigrant women found limited evidence for culturally sensitive or non-Western approaches to postpartum mental health (Fung & Dennis, 2010). A scoping review of theories, intergenerational pathways, interventions, and assessment tools for parents in the perinatal period with their own histories of childhood maltreatment found limited research, including Indigenous parents (Chamberlain et al., 2019). Family support and positive family relationships have been identified as one of the most prominent protective factors for perinatal mental health among Indigenous women (Carlin et al., 2021; Seear et al., 2021). Thus, in addition to collaborating with community members, the development and provision of perinatal support in diverse and Indigenous communities necessitate the inclusion of family and partners as best practice (Marriott & Kapetas, 2013). Future research is needed to inform how Indigenous ways of knowing may inform how to build resilience within the broader public health and healthcare systems.

System-Level Approaches

With nearly one in every three individuals having a history of child abuse (Afifi et al., 2014), consideration of how to address trauma and promote resilience in perinatal care should be universal (Racine et al., 2020).

Trauma-informed care (TIC) approaches consider the impact of trauma on health and employ supportive practices that actively avoid re-traumatization and promote healing in individuals exposed to trauma (Substance Abuse and Mental Health Services Administration, 2014). Within the perinatal setting, a TIC approach is relational and promotes compassionate, emotionally safe, trustworthy, and transparent care (Choi et al., 2020; Machtinger et al., 2015; Sperlich et al., 2017). In the prenatal setting, the integration of TIC is believed to facilitate supportive discussions about a history of child abuse, social support, and the safety of current relationships. Qualitative research with pregnant women and new mothers with trauma histories indicates that positive relationships, respect, and safety are key elements necessary in healthcare to increase comfort and trustworthiness with providers (Frederickson et al., 2022; Gokhale et al., 2020; Muzik et al., 2013).

Although the need for trauma-informed care is well described (Gokhale et al., 2020; Muzik et al., 2013), very few trauma-informed models and trauma-specific interventions have been developed for use with pregnancy and postpartum women (Sperlich et al., 2017). One study that did implement a TIC approach for pregnant women in primary care found increases in attendance at prenatal appointments and decreased rates of preterm birth compared to rates before the implementation of the TIC approach (Ashby et al., 2019). Another study demonstrated a slightly lower risk of infant birth complications for women who received a TIC approach than for women who did not (Racine et al., 2021). Taken together, TIC approaches are a promising universal approach to increasing resilience for women with child abuse histories. More research is needed to understand the mechanisms and long-term implications of TIC.

Conclusion

Research on the impact of child abuse on maternal physical and mental health during the perinatal period has demonstrated that these experiences are far from deterministic. In line with ecological systems theory, resilience occurs at multiple levels of the social ecology, including the individual, family, community, and system levels. Greater emphasis on approaches that extend beyond the individual, are culturally sensitive, and are trauma-informed holds the greatest promise for promoting positive outcomes. Research focused on understanding mechanisms and promoting the implementation of resilience-enhancing approaches within the perinatal setting is needed to advance understanding of how to build further resilience in the perinatal period for survivors of childhood abuse and adversity.

References

Afifi, T. O., MacMillan, H. L., Boyle, M., Taillieu, T., Cheung, K., & Sareen, J. (2014). Child abuse and mental disorders in Canada. *Canadian Medical Association Journal, 186*(9), E324–E332. https://doi.org/10.1503/cmaj.131792

Appleton, A. A., Kiley, K., Holdsworth, E. A., & Schell, L. M. (2019). Social support during pregnancy modifies the association between maternal adverse childhood experiences and infant birth size. *Maternal and Child Health Journal, 23*(3), 408–415. https://doi.org/10.1007/s10995-018-02706-z

Ashby, B. D., Ehmer, A. C., & Scott, S. M. (2019). Trauma-informed care in a patient-centered medical home for adolescent mothers and their children. *Psychological Services, 16*(1), 67–74. https://doi.org/10.1037/ser0000315

Atzl, V. M., Grande, L. A., Davis, E. P., & Narayan, A. J. (2019). Perinatal promotive and protective factors for women with histories of childhood abuse and neglect. *Child Abuse & Neglect, 91*, 63–77. https://doi.org/10.1016/j.chiabu.2019.02.008

Belsky, J., & Pluess, M. (2009). Beyond diathesis stress: Differential susceptibility to environmental influences. *Psychological Bulletin, 135*(6), 885–908. https://doi.org/10.1037/a0017376

Berthelot, N., Drouin-Maziade, C., Garon-Bissonnette, J., Lemieux, R., Series, T., & Lacharite, C. (2021). Evaluation of the acceptability of a prenatal program for women with histories of childhood trauma: The program STEP. *Frontiers in Psychiatry, 12*, 772706. https://doi.org/10.3389/fpsyt.2021.772706

Brunton, R., Wood, T., & Dryer, R. (2022). Childhood abuse, pregnancy-related anxiety and the mediating role of resilience and social support. *Journal of Health Psychology, 27*(4), 868–878. https://doi.org/10.1177/1359105320968140

Buultjens, M., Farouque, A., Karimi, L., Whitby, L., Milgrom, J., & Erbas, B. (2021). The contribution of group prenatal care to maternal psychological health outcomes: A systematic review. *Women and Birth, 34*(6), e631–e642. https://doi.org/10.1016/j.wombi.2020.12.004

Carlin, E., Seear, K. H., Ferrari, K., Spry, E., Atkinson, D., & Marley, J. V. (2021). Risk and resilience: A mixed methods investigation of aboriginal Australian women's perinatal mental health screening assessments. *Social Psychiatry and Psychiatric Epidemiology, 56*(4), 547–557. https://doi.org/10.1007/s00127-020-01986-7

Chamberlain, C., Gee, G., Harfield, S., Campbell, S., Brennan, S., Clark, Y., Mensah, F., Arabena, K., Herrman, H., & Brown, S. (2019). Parenting after a history of childhood maltreatment: A scoping review and map of evidence in the perinatal period. *PLoS One, 14*(3), e0213460. https://doi.org/10.1371/journal.pone.0213460

Choi, K. R., Records, K., Low, L. K., Alhusen, J. L., Kenner, C., Bloch, J. R., Premji, S. S., Hannan, J., Anderson, C. M., Yeo, S., & Cynthia Logsdon, M. (2020). Promotion of maternal-infant mental health and trauma-informed care during the COVID-19 pandemic. *Journal of Obstetric, Gynecologic, and Neonatal Nursing, 49*(5), 409–415. https://doi.org/10.1016/j.jogn.2020.07.004

Chung, E. K., Mathew, L., Elo, I. T., Coyne, J. C., & Culhane, J. F. (2008). Depressive symptoms in disadvantaged women receiving prenatal care: The influence of adverse and positive childhood experiences. *Ambulatory Pediatrics, 8*(2), 109–116. https://doi.org/10.1016/j.ambp.2007.12.003

Cooke, J. E., Racine, N., Pador, P., & Madigan, S. (2021). Maternal adverse childhood experiences and child behavior problems: A systematic review. *Pediatrics, 148*(3). https://doi.org/10.1542/peds.2020-044131

Folger, A. T., Eismann, E. A., Stephenson, N. B., Shapiro, R. A., Macaluso, M., Brownrigg, M. E., & Gillespie, R. J. (2018). Parental adverse childhood experiences and offspring development at 2 years of age. *Pediatrics, 141*(4). https://doi.org/10.1542/peds.2017-2826

Frederickson, A., Kern, A., & Langevin, R. (2022). Perinatal (re)experiencing of post-traumatic stress disorder symptoms for survivors of childhood sexual Abuse: An integrative review. *Journal of Women's Health, 32*(1), 78. https://doi.org/10.1089/jwh.2022.0183

Fung, K., & Dennis, C. L. (2010). Postpartum depression among immigrant women. *Current Opinion in Psychiatry, 23*(4), 342–348. https://doi.org/10.1097/YCO.0b013e32833ad721

Gokhale, P., Young, M. R., Williams, M. N., Reid, S. N., Tom, L. S., O'Brian, C. A., & Simon, M. A. (2020). Refining trauma-informed perinatal care for urban prenatal care patients with multiple lifetime traumatic exposures: A qualitative study. *Journal of Midwifery & Women's Health*, *65*(2), 224–230. https://doi.org/10.1111/jmwh.13063

Handford, P. (2011). *Postpartum depression and anxiety: A reference manual for group facilitation* (3rd ed.). Pacific Post Partum Support Society.

Howell, K. H., Miller-Graff, L. E., Martinez-Torteya, C., Napier, T. R., & Carney, J. R. (2021). Charting a course towards resilience following adverse childhood experiences: Addressing intergenerational trauma via strengths-based intervention. *Children (Basel)*, *8*(10). https://doi.org/10.3390/children8100844

Hudziak, J. J. (2018). ACEs and pregnancy: Time to support all expectant mothers. *Pediatrics*, *141*(4). https://doi.org/10.1542/peds.2018-0232

Hughes, K., Bellis, M. A., Hardcastle, K. A., Sethi, D., Butchart, A., Mikton, C., Jones, L., & Dunne, M. P. (2017). The effect of multiple adverse childhood experiences on health: A systematic review and meta-analysis. *The Lancet Public Health*, *2*(8), e356–e366. https://doi.org/10.1016/S2468-2667(17)30118-4

Kern, A., Frederickson, A., Hebert, M., Bernier, A., Frappier, J. Y., & Langevin, R. (2022a). Exploring the relationships between child maltreatment and risk factors for pregnancy complications. *Journal of Obstetrics and Gynaecology Canada*, *44*(5), 496–502. https://doi.org/10.1016/j.jogc.2021.11.013

Kern, A., Khoury, B., Frederickson, A., & Langevin, R. (2022b). The associations between childhood maltreatment and pregnancy complications: A systematic review and meta-analysis. *Journal of Psychosomatic Research*, *160*, 110985. https://doi.org/10.1016/j.jpsychores.2022.110985

Kershaw, K. N., Marsh, D. J., Crenshaw, E. G., McNeil, R. B., Pemberton, V. L., Cordon, S. A., Haas, D. M., Debbink, M. P., Mercer, B. M., Parry, S., Reddy, U., Saade, G., Simhan, H., Wapner, R. J., Wing, D. A., Grobman, W. A., & and for the NICHD nuMoM2b and NHLBI nuMoM2b Heart Health Study Networks. (2021). Associations of the neighborhood built environment with physical activity across pregnancy. *Journal of Physical Activity and Health*, *18*(5), 541–547. https://doi.org/10.1123/jpah.2020-0510

Kitzman, H., Olds, D. L., Sidora, K., Henderson, J. C. R., Hanks, C., Cole, R., Luckey, D. W., Bondy, J., Cole, K., & Glazner, J. (2000). Enduring effects of nurse home visitation on maternal life course. *JAMA*, *283*(15), 1983. https://doi.org/10.1001/jama.283.15.1983

Lebel, C., MacKinnon, A., Bagshawe, M., Tomfohr-Madsen, L., & Giesbrecht, G. (2020). Elevated depression and anxiety symptoms among pregnant individuals during the COVID-19 pandemic. *Journal of Affective Disorders, 277*, 5–13. https://doi.org/10.1016/j.jad.2020.07.126

Leeners, B., Stiller, R., Block, E., Gorres, G., & Rath, W. (2010). Pregnancy complications in women with childhood sexual abuse experiences. *Journal of Psychosomatic Research, 69*(5), 503–510. https://doi.org/10.1016/j.jpsychores.2010.04.017

Leigh, B., & Milgrom, J. (2008). Risk factors for antenatal depression, postnatal depression and parenting stress. *BMC Psychiatry, 8*, 24. https://doi.org/10.1186/1471-244X-8-24

Liu, Y., Wang, Y., Wu, Y., Chen, X., & Bai, J. (2021). Effectiveness of the CenteringPregnancy program on maternal and birth outcomes: A systematic review and meta-analysis. *International Journal of Nursing Studies, 120*, 103981. https://doi.org/10.1016/j.ijnurstu.2021.103981

Machtinger, E. L., Cuca, Y. P., Khanna, N., Rose, C. D., & Kimberg, L. S. (2015). From treatment to healing: The promise of trauma-informed primary care. *Women's Health Issues, 25*(3), 193–197. https://doi.org/10.1016/j.whi.2015.03.008

Madigan, S., Wade, M., Plamondon, A., & Jenkins, J. M. (2016). Neighborhood collective efficacy moderates the association between maternal adverse childhood experiences and marital conflict. *American Journal of Community Psychology, 57*(3–4), 437–447. https://doi.org/10.1002/ajcp.12053

Madigan, S., Wade, M., Plamondon, A., Maguire, J. L., & Jenkins, J. M. (2017). Maternal adverse childhood experience and infant health: Biomedical and psychosocial risks as intermediary mechanisms. *The Journal of Pediatrics, 187*, 282–289. e281.. https://doi.org/10.1016/j.jpeds.2017.04.052

Marriott, R., & Kapetas, J. (2013). Collaborating with a regional community for optimal aboriginal perinatal mental health, parenting, cultural wellbeing and resilience. *International Journal of Mental Health Nursing, 22*(1), 18. https://doi.org/10.1111/inm.12047

Masten, A. (2021). Resilience in developmental systems: Principles, pathways, and protective processes in research and practice. In M. Ungar (Ed.), *Multisystemic resilience: Adaptation and transformation in contexts of change* (pp. 113–134). Oxford University Press.

Masten, A. S. (2013). Risk and resilience in development. In P. Zelazo (Ed.), *The Oxford handbook of developmental psychology* (Vol. 2. Self and other, pp. 579–607). Oxford University Press.

Maxwell, D., Robinson, S. R., & Rogers, K. (2019). "I keep it to myself": A qualitative meta-interpretive synthesis of experiences of postpartum depression among marginalised women. *Health and Social Care Community, 27*(3), e23–e36. https://doi.org/10.1111/hsc.12645

Mersky, J. P., & Lee, C. P. (2019). Adverse childhood experiences and poor birth outcomes in a diverse, low-income sample. *BMC Pregnancy and Childbirth, 19*(1), 387. https://doi.org/10.1186/s12884-019-2560-8

Miller, E. S., Fleming, O., Ekpe, E. E., Grobman, W. A., & Heard-Garris, N. (2021). Association between adverse childhood experiences and adverse pregnancy outcomes. *Obstetrics & Gynecology, 138*(5), 770–776. https://doi.org/10.1097/AOG.0000000000004570

Muzik, M., Ads, M., Bonham, C., Lisa Rosenblum, K., Broderick, A., & Kirk, R. (2013). Perspectives on trauma-informed care from mothers with a history of childhood maltreatment: A qualitative study. *Child Abuse & Neglect, 37*(12), 1215–1224. https://doi.org/10.1016/j.chiabu.2013.07.014

Narayan, A. J., Lieberman, A. F., & Masten, A. S. (2021). Intergenerational transmission and prevention of adverse childhood experiences (ACEs). *Clinical Psychology Review, 85*, 101997. https://doi.org/10.1016/j.cpr.2021.101997

Narayan, A. J., Rivera, L. M., Bernstein, R. E., Harris, W. W., & Lieberman, A. F. (2018). Positive childhood experiences predict less psychopathology and stress in pregnant women with childhood adversity: A pilot study of the benevolent childhood experiences (BCEs) scale. *Child Abuse & Neglect, 78*, 19–30. https://doi.org/10.1016/j.chiabu.2017.09.022

Olds, D. L. (2006). The nurse-family partnership: An evidence-based preventive intervention. *Infant Mental Health Journal, 27*(1), 5–25. https://doi.org/10.1002/imhj.20077

Olds, D. L., Henderson, C. R., Tatelbaum, R., & Chamberlin, R. (1986). Improving the delivery of prenatal care and outcomes of pregnancy: A randomized trial of nurse home visitation. *Pediatrics, 77*(1), 16–28.

Olsen, J. M. (2018). Integrative review of pregnancy health risks and outcomes associated with adverse childhood experiences. *Journal of Obstetric, Gynecologic & Neonatal Nursing, 47*(6), 783–794.

Osofsky, J. D., Osofsky, H. J., Frazer, A. L., Fields-Olivieri, M. A., Many, M., Selby, M., Holman, S., & Conrad, E. (2021). The importance of adverse childhood experiences during the perinatal period. *American Psychologist, 76*(2), 350–363. https://doi.org/10.1037/amp0000770

Racine, N., Ereyi-Osas, W., Killam, T., McDonald, S., & Madigan, S. (2021). Maternal-child health outcomes from pre- to post-implementation of a trauma-informed care initiative in the prenatal care setting: A retrospective study. *Children (Basel), 8*(11). https://doi.org/10.3390/children8111061

Racine, N., Killam, T., & Madigan, S. (2020). Trauma-informed care as a universal precaution: Beyond the adverse childhood experiences questionnaire. *JAMA Pediatrics, 174*(1), 5–6. https://doi.org/10.1001/jamapediatrics.2019.3866

Racine, N., Madigan, S., Plamondon, A., Hetherington, E., McDonald, S., & Tough, S. (2018a). Maternal adverse childhood experiences and antepartum risks: The moderating role of social support. *Archives of Women's Mental Health, 21*(6), 663–670. https://doi.org/10.1007/s00737-018-0826-1

Racine, N., Plamondon, A., Hentges, R., Tough, S., & Madigan, S. (2019). Dynamic and bidirectional associations between maternal stress, anxiety, and social support: The critical role of partner and family support. *Journal of Affective Disorders, 252*, 19–24. https://doi.org/10.1016/j.jad.2019.03.083

Racine, N., Plamondon, A., Madigan, S., McDonald, S., & Tough, S. (2018b). Maternal adverse childhood experiences and infant development. *Pediatrics, 141*(4), e20172495. https://doi.org/10.1542/peds.2017-2495

Rowe, H., Sperlich, M., Cameron, H., & Seng, J. (2014). A quasi-experimental outcomes analysis of a psychoeducation intervention for pregnant women with abuse-related posttraumatic stress. *Journal of Obstetric, Gynecologic & Neonatal Nursing, 43*(3), 282–293. https://doi.org/10.1111/1552-6909.12312

Seear, K. H., Spry, E. P., Carlin, E., Atkinson, D. N., & Marley, J. V. (2021). Aboriginal women's experiences of strengths and challenges of antenatal care in the Kimberley: A qualitative study. *Women and Birth, 34*(6), 570–577. https://doi.org/10.1016/j.wombi.2020.12.009

Sexton, M. B., Hamilton, L., McGinnis, E. W., Rosenblum, K. L., & Muzik, M. (2015). The roles of resilience and childhood trauma history: Main and moderating effects on postpartum maternal mental health and functioning. *Journal of Affective Disorders, 174*, 562–568. https://doi.org/10.1016/j.jad.2014.12.036

Smith, M. V., Gotman, N., & Yonkers, K. A. (2016). Early childhood adversity and pregnancy outcomes. *Maternal and Child Health Journal, 20*(4), 790–798. https://doi.org/10.1007/s10995-015-1909-5

Sperlich, M., & Seng, J. (2018). Survivor mom's companion: A population-level program for pregnant women who are survivors of childhood maltreatment:

The need for a public health approach to addressing unresolved maternal trauma. In M. Muzik & K. Rosenblum (Eds.), *Motherhood in the face of trauma. Integrating psychiatry and primary care.* Springer. https://doi.org/10.1007/978-3-319-65724-0_13

Sperlich, M., Seng, J. S., Li, Y., Taylor, J., & Bradbury-Jones, C. (2017). Integrating trauma-informed care into maternity care practice: Conceptual and practical issues. *Journal of Midwifery & Women's Health, 62*(6), 661–672. https://doi.org/10.1111/jmwh.12674

Substance Abuse and Mental Health Services Administration. (2014). *SAMHSA's concept of trauma and guidance for a trauma-informed approach.*

Thomas, J. C., Letourneau, N., Campbell, T. S., Giesbrecht, G. F., & Apron Study, T. (2018). Social buffering of the maternal and infant HPA axes: Mediation and moderation in the intergenerational transmission of adverse childhood experiences. *Development and Psychopathology, 30*(3), 921–939. https://doi.org/10.1017/S0954579418000512

Thornberry, T. P., Henry, K. L., Smith, C. A., Ireland, T. O., Greenman, S. J., & Lee, R. D. (2013). Breaking the cycle of maltreatment: The role of safe, stable, and nurturing relationships. *Journal of Adolescent Health, 53*(4), S25–S31. https://doi.org/10.1016/j.jadohealth.2013.04.019

Ungar, M., Ghazinour, M., & Richter, J. (2013). Annual research review: What is resilience within the social ecology of human development? *Journal of Child Psychology and Psychiatry, 54*(4), 348–366. https://doi.org/10.1111/jcpp.12025

Vinikoor-Imler, L. C., Messer, L. C., Evenson, K. R., & Laraia, B. A. (2011). Neighborhood conditions are associated with maternal health behaviors and pregnancy outcomes. *Social Science & Medicine, 73*(9), 1302–1311. https://doi.org/10.1016/j.socscimed.2011.08.012

Xuemei, M., Wang, Y., Hu, H., Tao, X. G., Zhang, Y., & Shi, H. (2019). The impact of resilience on prenatal anxiety and depression among pregnant women in Shanghai. *Journal of Affective Disorders, 250*, 57–64. https://doi.org/10.1016/j.jad.2019.02.058

Young-Wolff, K. C., Alabaster, A., McCaw, B., Stoller, N., Watson, C., Sterling, S., Ridout, K. K., & Flanagan, T. (2019). Adverse childhood experiences and mental and behavioral health conditions during pregnancy: The role of resilience. *Journal of Women's Health (2002), 28*(4), 452–461. https://doi.org/10.1089/jwh.2018.7108

9

Conclusion

Rachel Dryer ⓘ and Robyn Brunton ⓘ

Abstract In this final chapter, our aim was to reflect on the important ideas emerging from the chapters in this book. A summary of the ideas contained in each chapter is presented along with identification of the common themes presented by the authors. A core theme that arose from the majority of chapters is that of pregnancy being a 'critical period' during which healthcare professionals and clinicians have the valuable opportunity to assist in resolving unresolved maternal trauma in individuals with child abuse histories before they become parents. The provision of (a) the opportunity to resolve maternal trauma and (b) trauma-informed

R. Dryer (✉)
School of Behavioural & Health Sciences (Faculty of Health Science),
Australian Catholic University, Strathfield, NSW, Australia
e-mail: rachel.dryer@acu.edu.au

R. Brunton
School of Psychology, Charles Sturt University, Bathurst, NSW, Australia
e-mail: rbrunton@csu.edu.au

R. Brunton, R. Dryer (eds.), *Perinatal Care and Considerations for Survivors of Child Abuse*, https://doi.org/10.1007/978-3-031-33639-3_9

perinatal care to avoid re-traumatization was regarded as key to better well-being outcomes for pregnant individuals with child abuse histories. Lastly, we propose a structured model on the determinants of well-being of child abuse survivors that pulled together the important thoughts presented by the chapter authors.

Keywords Pregnancy • Unresolved trauma • Trauma-informed perinatal care • Multi-level determinants of care

The main objective of this book is to provide a comprehensive source text for mental health professionals, clinicians, researchers, educators, and postgraduate students. We have achieved this by getting prominent clinicians and researchers to provide a multidisciplinary perspective of the current and emerging literature on maternal child abuse experience and perinatal outcomes for the childbearing individual and their infant. Each clinician/researcher examined a key issue with regards to the theoretical foundations, empirical research, or application. Their willingness to be involved in this book demonstrates their passion and drive to advance knowledge and practice on how best to promote well-being in the delivery of perinatal care.

In this final chapter, our aim is to consider the important ideas emerging from the chapters in this book. We will first summarize the ideas presented in each chapter and then identify the common themes presented by the authors. Lastly, we will propose a structured model on the determinants of well-being of child abuse survivors that pulls together the important thoughts presented by the authors.

In Chaps. 2 (Brunton) and 3 (Brunton & Dryer), the authors provide a theoretical foundation for the book by discussing the issues surrounding defining child abuse and how differences in definition and a lack of definitional consensus and recognition of the different types of abuse can affect prevalence estimates reported in the research and gray literature. An examination of the six key theoretical frameworks for maternal child abuse and its potential sequelae for childbearing individuals highlights that while the models have varying limitations in their application to perinatal research, they all have the potential to explain the outcomes related to child abuse histories during the perinatal period. It is noteworthy that the subsequent, more empirically focused chapters (Chaps. 4, 5, and 6) refer to the cumulative effects of adversity on well-being for both the childbearing individual and their infant, which is in line with the developmental cascade theories of child abuse.

In Chap. 4, Seng provides a comprehensive biopsychosocial overview of post-traumatic stress disorder (PTSD) and complex PTSD in pregnant individuals with child abuse histories. Svelnys and colleagues (Chap. 5) apply a developmental psychopathology perspective on the pathway between child abuse histories and psychological distress (i.e., anxiety and depression) and suicidal thoughts/behaviors. The authors of both chapters advocate trauma-informed care principles for the training of healthcare professionals, screening for child abuse histories, and the delivery of supports and interventions. As described by Seng, trauma-informed care practices will allow healthcare professionals and clinicians to "realize, recognize and respond" to victims of child abuse while minimizing the risk of retraumatizing them. These sentiments are echoed by Sperlich and Mendel in their examination of both client- and provider-level barriers to screening for child abuse histories in the delivery of perinatal care services (Chap. 7). While screening provides opportunities to identify child abuse survivors and address unresolved maternal trauma during pregnancy, these authors argue that the conditions under which such screening can occur need to be trauma-informed to avoid re-traumatization of victims, and where screening is conducted as part of a continuum of trauma responsivity that includes trauma-informed training for healthcare professionals, preparation, screening, referral to services and supports, and intervention. Trauma-informed care practices are also advocated by Racine and colleagues (Chap. 8) in their examination of how to promote resilience in individuals with child abuse histories during the perinatal period.

The majority of chapter authors (i.e., Brunton, Chap. 2; Seng, Chap. 4; Svelnys and colleagues, Chap. 5; Mohler & Brunton, Chap. 6; Sperlich & Mendel, Chap. 7; and Racine and colleagues, Chap. 8) see pregnancy as a 'critical period' during which healthcare professionals and clinicians can help resolve unresolved maternal trauma in individuals with child abuse histories before they become parents. The provision of (a) the opportunity to resolve maternal trauma and (b) trauma-informed perinatal care to avoid re-traumatization is regarded as key to better well-being outcomes for pregnant individuals with child abuse histories.

The authors of the chapters in this book identify some gaps in the current literature. Brunton (Chap. 1) argues that failure to recognize comorbidity of abuse types and assuming equivalence of risk among abuse types limit our understanding of the impact of maternal child abuse on perinatal well-being. Brunton advocates for controlling for the different abuse types in this research. Seng (Chap. 4) identifies a significant gap in research involving culturally diverse individuals despite PTSD and negative birth outcomes occurring at much higher rates for cultural groups that experience racism, discrimination, and marginalization. Similarly, Svelnys and colleagues (Chap. 5) advocate for the expansion of research to include gender-diverse individuals and their non-gestational partners whose pregnancy journey will be different to cisgender and heterosexual women, as well as gender-diverse individuals who experience discrimination and marginalization in society and higher rates of psychological distress and suicide risk (Ralston et al., 2022; Taylor et al., 2020). Svelnys and colleagues also highlight that much of the current research has primarily focused on well-being outcomes for women with live births, and that there is limited research on individuals with child abuse histories who have experienced termination of pregnancy (miscarriage, abortion, fetal, or infant death). They argue that this narrow focus limits our understanding of whether child abuse histories and perinatal mental health problems are associated with reproductive or fertility problems. Mohler and Brunton (Chap. 6) identified a need for more research examining child abuse histories and its influence on maternal-fetal attachment, a key developmental task of pregnancy which can affect postnatal behavior and bonding. Addressing these gaps in research will lead to a better understanding of the mechanisms that underlie the development and maintenance of negative physical and psychological well-being outcomes and suicide risk for survivors of child abuse as they navigate pregnancy and parenthood.

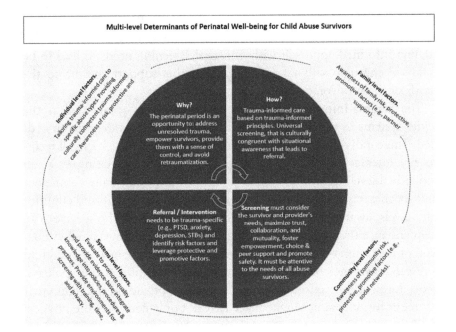

Fig. 9.1 Multi-level determinants of perinatal well-being for child abuse survivors

Figure 9.1 presents the Multi-level Determinants of Perinatal Well-Being for Child Abuse Survivors. As shown, the model depicts the multiple levels that may reciprocally affect the well-being of perinatal child abuse survivors. The model shows the opportunities that the perinatal period affords to address unresolved trauma, provide empowerment to survivors and a sense of control, and, importantly, avoid re-traumatization. This is done within the principles of trauma-informed care that include culturally congruent universal screening for trauma that requires situational awareness for privacy and confidentiality and must consider the needs of both the survivor and provider. Integral to screening are principles of trust, collaboration, and mutuality that help to foster empowerment for the survivor and above all promote physical and psychological safety. The screening also needs to be attentive to the needs of all abuse survivors, such as those who may have suffered physical abuse, psychological abuse, or multi-type maltreatment. And finally, this trauma-informed approach with universal screening needs to lead to be followed through with referral to intervention/support specific to the needs of the survivor.

The trauma-informed approach advocated here occurs within the wider systems in which individuals and healthcare providers are embedded. These individual, family, community, and system levels can all reciprocally interact on the well-being of the survivor. For example, at an individual level, trauma-informed care needs to be culturally competent and specific to the experience of the survivor. At the family and community levels, awareness of specific factors that can affect the survivor can help enhance their experience perinatally. And at a systems level, evaluation of the trauma-informed response will promote the quality and build a research evidence base to allow integration into more formal policies, procedures, and practices. Important to this is providing the right environment for screening to take place that not only considers the physical aspects of that environment but also provides appropriate training, support, and workload for those providing the screening.

The Multi-level Determinants of Perinatal Well-Being for Child Abuse Survivors model provides a framework for clinicians. Importantly this model can also be useful for research to address significant gaps in the literature that pertain to how to best support survivors of abuse. Sperlich and Mendel (Chap. 7) advocate for more research in evaluating the effectiveness of supports and interventions for pregnant individuals with child abuse histories, particularly trauma-specific interventions to address PTSD and depression. Likewise, Racine and colleagues (Chap. 8) identify a need for more research on developing and evaluating interventions and supports (at an individual level, family level, community level, and system level) that are culturally safe and trauma informed. Therefore, despite the diverse breadth of research reported in the various chapters of this book, the gaps in current research indicate that there is still significant work that needs to be done to advance our understanding of maternal child abuse and perinatal outcomes.

References

Ralston, A. L., Holt, N. R., Andrews, A. R., Huit, T. Z., Puckett, J. A., Woodruff, N., Mocarski, R., & Hope, D. A. (2022). Mental health and marginalization stress in transgender and gender diverse adults: Differences between urban and non-urban experiences. *Psychology of Sexual Orientation and Gender Diversity*. https://doi.org/10.1037/sgd0000595

Taylor, J., Power, J., Smith, E., & Rathbone, M. (2020). Bisexual mental health and gender diversity: Findings from the "Who I Am" study. *Australian Journal of General Practice, 49*(7), 392–399. https://doi.org/10.31128/AJGP-09-19-5073

Index[1]

---

[1] Note: Page numbers followed by 'n' refer to notes.

Printed in the USA
CPSIA information can be obtained
at www.ICGtesting.com
LVHW011954160324
774517LV00004B/407